Health Literacy in Clinical Research

Practice and Impact

PROCEEDINGS OF A WORKSHOP

Alexis Wojtowicz and Melissa G. French, *Rapporteurs*

Roundtable on Health Literacy

Board on Population Health and Public Health Practice

Health and Medicine Division

The National Academies of
SCIENCES · ENGINEERING · MEDICINE

THE NATIONAL ACADEMIES PRESS
Washington, DC
www.nap.edu

THE NATIONAL ACADEMIES PRESS 500 Fifth Street, NW Washington, DC 20001

This activity was supported by contracts between the National Academy of Sciences and AbbVie Inc.; California Dental Association; East Bay Community Foundation (Kaiser Permanente); Eli Lilly and Company; Health Literacy Media; Health Literacy Partners; Health Resources and Services Administration (HHSH25034011T); Merck Sharp & Dohme Corp.; National Library of Medicine; Northwell Health; Office of Disease Prevention and Health Promotion (HHSP23337043); Pfizer Inc.; and UnitedHealth Group. Any opinions, findings, conclusions, or recommendations expressed in this publication do not necessarily reflect the views of any organization or agency that provided support for the project.

International Standard Book Number-13: 978-0-309-49969-9
International Standard Book Number-10: 0-309-49969-0
Digital Object Identifier: https://doi.org/10.17226/25616

Additional copies of this publication are available from the National Academies Press, 500 Fifth Street, NW, Keck 360, Washington, DC 20001; (800) 624-6242 or (202) 334-3313; http://www.nap.edu.

Copyright 2020 by the National Academy of Sciences. All rights reserved.

Printed in the United States of America

Suggested citation: National Academies of Sciences, Engineering, and Medicine. 2020. *Health literacy in clinical research: Practice and impact: Proceedings of a workshop*. Washington, DC: The National Academies Press. https://doi.org/10.17226/25616.

The National Academies of
SCIENCES · ENGINEERING · MEDICINE

The **National Academy of Sciences** was established in 1863 by an Act of Congress, signed by President Lincoln, as a private, nongovernmental institution to advise the nation on issues related to science and technology. Members are elected by their peers for outstanding contributions to research. Dr. Marcia McNutt is president.

The **National Academy of Engineering** was established in 1964 under the charter of the National Academy of Sciences to bring the practices of engineering to advising the nation. Members are elected by their peers for extraordinary contributions to engineering. Dr. John L. Anderson is president.

The **National Academy of Medicine** (formerly the Institute of Medicine) was established in 1970 under the charter of the National Academy of Sciences to advise the nation on medical and health issues. Members are elected by their peers for distinguished contributions to medicine and health. Dr. Victor J. Dzau is president.

The three Academies work together as the **National Academies of Sciences, Engineering, and Medicine** to provide independent, objective analysis and advice to the nation and conduct other activities to solve complex problems and inform public policy decisions. The National Academies also encourage education and research, recognize outstanding contributions to knowledge, and increase public understanding in matters of science, engineering, and medicine.

Learn more about the National Academies of Sciences, Engineering, and Medicine at **www.nationalacademies.org**.

The National Academies of
SCIENCES · ENGINEERING · MEDICINE

Consensus Study Reports published by the National Academies of Sciences, Engineering, and Medicine document the evidence-based consensus on the study's statement of task by an authoring committee of experts. Reports typically include findings, conclusions, and recommendations based on information gathered by the committee and the committee's deliberations. Each report has been subjected to a rigorous and independent peer-review process, and it represents the position of the National Academies on the statement of task.

Proceedings published by the National Academies of Sciences, Engineering, and Medicine chronicle the presentations and discussions at a workshop, symposium, or other event convened by the National Academies. The statements and opinions contained in proceedings are those of the participants and are not endorsed by other participants, the planning committee, or the National Academies.

For information about other products and activities of the National Academies, please visit www.nationalacademies.org/about/whatwedo.

PLANNING COMMITTEE ON HEALTH LITERACY IN CLINICAL TRIALS: PRACTICE AND IMPACT[1]

ANNLOUISE R. ASSAF, Patient Health Activation Expert and Global Medical Impact Assessment Senior Director, Pfizer Worldwide Medical and Safety; Professor (Adjunct), Brown University School of Public Health

BARBARA E. BIERER, Professor of Medicine and Faculty Director, Multi-Regional Clinical Trials Center of Brigham and Women's Hospital and Harvard

TERRY C. DAVIS, Professor of Medicine and Pediatrics, Louisiana State University Health Sciences Center–Shreveport

LAUREN McCORMACK, Vice President, Public Health Research Division, RTI International

LAURIE MYERS, Global Health Literacy Director, Merck Sharp & Dohme Corp.

CATINA O'LEARY, President and Chief Executive Officer, Health Literacy Media

PHYLLIS J. PETTIT NASSI, Associate Director, Research and Science, Special Populations, American Indian Program, University of Utah Huntsman Cancer Institute

PATTY SPEARS, Research Patient Advocate, University of North Carolina Lineberger Comprehensive Cancer Center

CONSUELO H. WILKINS, Vice President for Health Equity, Vanderbilt University Medical Center

---

[1] The National Academies of Sciences, Engineering, and Medicine's planning committees are solely responsible for organizing the workshop, identifying topics, and choosing speakers. The responsibility for the published Proceedings of a Workshop rests with the workshop rapporteurs and the institution.

ROUNDTABLE ON HEALTH LITERACY[1]

LAWRENCE G. SMITH (*Chair*), Dean, Donald and Barbara Zucker School of Medicine at Hofstra/Northwell; Executive Vice President and Physician-in-Chief, Northwell Health

ANNLOUISE R. ASSAF, Patient Health Activation Expert and Global Medical Impact Assessment Senior Director, Pfizer Worldwide Medical and Safety; Professor (Adjunct), Brown University School of Public Health

SUZANNE BAKKEN, Alumni Professor of Nursing and Professor of Biomedical Informatics, Columbia University

GEMIRALD DAUS, Public Health Analyst, Office of Health Equity, Health Resources and Services Administration

TERRY C. DAVIS, Professor of Medicine and Pediatrics, Louisiana State University Health Sciences Center–Shreveport

JENNIFER DILLAHA, Medical Director for Immunizations, Medical Advisor, Health Literacy and Communication, Arkansas Department of Health

JAMES DUHIG, Head, Risk Communication and Behavioral Systems, Office of Patient Safety, AbbVie Inc.

ALICIA FERNÁNDEZ, Professor of Medicine, Director, UCSF Latinx Center of Excellence, University of California, San Francisco, Zuckerberg San Francisco General Hospital

LISA FITZPATRICK, Senior Medical Director, DC Department of Health Care Finance, and Professorial Lecturer, The George Washington Milken Institute of Public Health

LORI K. HALL, Director of Health Literacy, Global Medical Strategy and Operations, Eli Lilly and Company

LINDA HARRIS, Director, Division of Health Communication and eHealth Team, Office of Disease Prevention and Health Promotion, U.S. Department of Health and Human Services

NICOLE HOLLAND, Assistant Professor and Director of Health Communication, Education, and Promotion, Tufts University School of Dental Medicine

ELLEN MARKMAN, Lewis M. Terman Professor of Psychology, Stanford University

JOHANNA MARTINEZ, Graduate Medical Education Director of Diversity and Health Equity, Northwell Health

---

[1] The National Academies of Sciences, Engineering, and Medicine's forums and roundtables do not issue, review, or approve individual documents. The responsibility for the published Proceedings of a Workshop rests with the workshop rapporteurs and the institution.

MICHAEL McKEE, Associate Professor of Family Medicine, Director of MDisability, University of Michigan Medical School
LAURIE MYERS, Global Health Literacy Director, Merck Sharp & Dohme Corp.
CATINA O'LEARY, President and Chief Executive Officer, Health Literacy Media
MICHAEL PAASCHE-ORLOW, Professor of Medicine, Boston University School of Medicine
TERRI ANN PARNELL, Principal and Founder, Health Literacy Partners
LINDSEY A. ROBINSON, Diplomate, ABPD, California Dental Association
STEVEN RUSH, Director, Health Literacy Innovations, UnitedHealth Group
OLAYINKA SHIYANBOLA, Assistant Professor, Division of Social and Administrative Sciences, University of Wisconsin–Madison School of Pharmacy
VANESSA SIMONDS, Assistant Professor, Community Health, Montana State University
CHRISTOPHER R. TRUDEAU, Associate Professor of Medical Humanities, University of Arkansas for Medical Sciences; Associate Professor of Law, Bowen School of Law, University of Arkansas at Little Rock
EARNESTINE WILLIS, Kellner Professor in Pediatrics, Medical College of Wisconsin
AMANDA J. WILSON, Head, Engagement and Training, National Library of Medicine
MICHAEL S. WOLF, Professor, Medicine and Learning Sciences, Associate Division Chief, Research Division of General Internal Medicine, Feinberg School of Medicine, Northwestern University
WINSTON F. WONG, Medical Director, Disparities Improvement and Quality Initiatives, Kaiser Permanente

Health and Medicine Division Staff

MELISSA G. FRENCH, Senior Program Officer (*until January 2020*)
ALEXIS WOJTOWICZ, Research Associate
ANNA W. MARTIN, Administrative Assistant
ROSE MARIE MARTINEZ, Senior Board Director, Board on Population Health and Public Health Practice

Reviewers

This Proceedings of a Workshop was reviewed in draft form by individuals chosen for their diverse perspectives and technical expertise. The purpose of this independent review is to provide candid and critical comments that will assist the National Academies of Sciences, Engineering, and Medicine in making each published proceedings as sound as possible and to ensure that it meets the institutional standards for quality, objectivity, evidence, and responsiveness to the charge. The review comments and draft manuscript remain confidential to protect the integrity of the process.

We thank the following individuals for their review of this proceedings:

CONNIE CITRO, Division of Behavioral and Social Sciences and Education, The National Academies of Sciences, Engineering, and Medicine

SYLVIA BAEDORF KASSIS, Multi-Regional Clinical Trials Center of Brigham and Women's Hospital and Harvard

Although the reviewers listed above provided many constructive comments and suggestions, they were not asked to endorse the content of the proceedings nor did they see the final draft before its release. The review of this proceedings was overseen by **DEBORAH E. POWELL,** University of Minnesota Medical School. She was responsible for making certain that an independent examination of this proceedings was carried out in accordance with standards of the National Academies and that all review comments were carefully considered. Responsibility for the final content rests entirely with the rapporteurs and the National Academies.

Acknowledgments

The sponsors of the Roundtable on Health Literacy made it possible to plan and conduct the workshop Health Literacy in Clinical Trials: Practice and Impact, which this proceedings summarizes. Federal sponsors from the U.S. Department of Health and Human Services are the Health Resources and Services Administration; National Library of Medicine; and Office of Disease Prevention and Health Promotion. Nonfederal sponsorship was provided by AbbVie Inc.; California Dental Association; East Bay Community Foundation (Kaiser Permanente); Eli Lilly and Company; Health Literacy Media; Health Literacy Partners; Merck Sharp & Dohme Corp.; Northwell Health; Pfizer Inc.; and UnitedHealth Group.

The workshop presentations were interesting and stimulated much discussion, and the Roundtable on Health Literacy would like to thank each of the speakers and moderators for their time and effort. Speakers and moderators were Emma Andrews, Connie Arnold, Annlouise R. Assaf, Barbara E. Bierer, Ebony Boulware, Deborah Collyar, Terry C. Davis, Lauren McCormack, Monika Mitra, Catina O'Leary, Phyllis J. Pettit Nassi, Saira Z. Sheikh, Lawrence G. Smith, Patty Spears, Jovonni R. Spinner, Alicia Staley, Christopher R. Trudeau, Consuelo H. Wilkins, and Rebecca J. Williams.

Contents

ACRONYMS AND ABBREVIATIONS   xvii

1   INTRODUCTION   1
Organization of the Proceedings, 3

2   HEALTH LITERACY AS AN ETHICAL IMPERATIVE
IN CLINICAL TRIALS   5
Why Health Literacy Matters, 5
Health Literacy Helps Patients Make Decisions:
    A Patient Perspective, 11
Discussion, 17
References, 21

3   EMBEDDING HEALTH LITERACY IN CLINICAL
TRIALS TO IMPROVE RECRUITMENT
AND RETENTION   23
Enrolling Minorities with Variable Literacy in Clinical Trials, 24
Lessons Learned from Behavioral Trials of African Americans, 26
Health-Literate Materials for Recruitment and Retention, 27
Technological Tools to Improve Patient Experiences, 31
Regulatory Changes in Clinical Trials, 33
Discussion, 35
References, 46

4	EXPERIENCES IMPLEMENTING HEALTH LITERACY BEST PRACTICES IN CLINICAL TRIALS	49

Lessons Learned from Two Health Literacy Interventions
 to Improve Colorectal Cancer Screenings, 49
Making Clinical Trials and Informed Consent More
 Patient-Centered, 54
Critical Conversations in Clinical Trials, 58
Discussion, 63
References, 66

5	DESIGNING CLINICAL TRIALS WITH HEALTH LITERACY BEST PRACTICES	69

Presentations, 69
Discussion, 76
References, 80

6	REFLECTIONS, RESEARCH DIRECTIONS, AND POTENTIAL OPPORTUNITIES FOR IMPLEMENTATION	81

Rapporteur Presentations, 81
Roundtable Discussion, 83
Reference, 86

APPENDIXES

A	Workshop Agenda	87
B	Biographical Sketches of Workshop Moderators, Speakers, and Panelists	91

Boxes, Figure, and Tables

BOXES

1-1 Statement of Task, 2

2-1 Possible Patient Questions Regarding Clinical Trials, 15

3-1 Key Points Raised by Individual Panelists, 24

4-1 Current Challenges Related to Informed Consent, 54
4-2 Strategies for Creating a Health-Literate Clinical Trials Environment, 63

6-1 Highlights from Rapporteur Presentations, 82
6-2 Key Observations from Roundtable Members, 84

A-1 Workshop Objectives and Questions, 87

FIGURE

3-1 Health literacy through the clinical trials process, 28

TABLES

2-1 Words Matter: Differences in Medical/Scientific Terms Among Medical Professionals Compared with the General Public, 13

3-1 Three Small Clinical Trials with African American Participants, 27

Acronyms and Abbreviations

AE	adverse event
AI/AN	American Indian/Alaska Native
CARE	Committee on Advocacy, Research Communication, Ethics, and Disparities
CEO	chief executive officer
CRC	colorectal cancer
CTSA	Clinical Translational Science Awards (NIH)
CTTI	Clinical Trials Transformation Initiative
CV	curriculum vitae
eIC	electronic informed consent
EMA	European Medicines Agency
EU	European Union
FDA	U.S. Food and Drug Administration
FIT	fecal immunochemical test
FOBT	fecal occult blood test
FQHC	federally qualified health center
GDPR	General Data Protection Regulation (European Union)
HIPAA	Health Insurance Portability and Accountability Act
HLM	Health Literacy Media

IRB	Institutional Review Board
LSU	Louisiana State University
MIMICT	Materials to Increase Minority Involvement in Clinical Trials
MRCT Center	Multi-Regional Clinical Trials Center of Brigham and Women's Hospital and Harvard
NIH	National Institutes of Health
NLM	National Library of Medicine
OMHHE	Office of Minority Health and Health Equity
PAIR	Patient Advocates in Research
PALS	Patient Advocates for Lupus Studies
PCP	primary care physician or primary care provider
PRO	patient-reported outcome
PSA	public service announcement
PURPLE	Programs to Address Unmet Needs and Promote Representation of All Participants in Lupus Clinical Trials Using Mobile Technology for Engagement
PWD	people with disabilities
RA	research assistant
REMS	risk evaluation and mitigation strategies
RIC	Recruitment Innovation Center
SACHRP	Secretary's Advisory Committee on Human Research Protections
UNC	University of North Carolina
WHI	Women's Health Initiative

1

Introduction[1]

The Roundtable on Health Literacy convened a workshop titled Clinical Trials: Practice and Impact on April 11, 2019, in Washington, DC. The workshop planning committee invited speakers and audience members to discuss the following topics:

1. Why are health literacy practices important for clinical trials?
2. What is the state of the science for incorporating health literacy practices into the design and execution of clinical trials?
3. How can health literacy improve the quality and outcomes of clinical trials?
4. What are the challenges and best practices for incorporating health literacy into clinical trials?

The workshop's complete Statement of Task can be found in Box 1-1 and the agenda can be found in Appendix A.

Clinical trials serve as the bedrock of successful diagnostic, preventive, and treatment interventions, and can serve patients experiencing any stage of a condition, disease, or syndrome. Those who participate in clinical trials provide a great service to the broader medical community because, through

---

[1] The planning committee's role was limited to planning the workshop, and the Proceedings of a Workshop was prepared by the workshop rapporteurs as a factual summary of what occurred at this workshop. Statements, recommendations, and opinions expressed are those of individual presenters and participants, and are not necessarily endorsed or verified by the National Academies of Sciences, Engineering, and Medicine, and they should not be construed as reflecting any group consensus.

> BOX 1-1
> Statement of Task
>
> An ad hoc planning committee will plan and conduct a 1-day public workshop that will feature invited presentations and discussion of incorporating health literacy principles into clinical trials. The workshop may include presentations and discussion of issues related to the challenges or barriers for diverse populations' participation in clinical trials, best practices for clinical trial sites and researchers incorporating health literacy practices, effective health literacy strategies for clear communication with participants, and other areas as appropriate. The planning committee will define the specific topics to be addressed, develop the agenda, select and invite speakers and other participants, and moderate the discussions. Proceedings of the presentations and discussions at the workshop will be developed by a designated rapporteur in accordance with institutional guidelines.

their willingness to experience the benefits and risks of a clinical trial's intervention, they help the medical community develop drugs and therapies that are most helpful to patients. However, because of the individualized nature of drug and therapeutic treatments, clinical trials require participants who represent the diversity of the patient base. If early trials do not have a broad patient base, it can be difficult to know who may or may not benefit from or respond to a treatment later. In addition to diversity in recruitment, informed consent during participation is also crucial. If participants do not fully understand what they are signing up for, they may become confused, mistrustful, or drop out of a trial altogether, confusing investigators and possibly affecting the generalizability of a study.

The workshop was opened by Lawrence G. Smith, dean of the Donald and Barbara Zucker School of Medicine at Hofstra/Northwell and physician-in-chief at Northwell Health, who offered some observations to set the stage for the day. "Many people who enroll in clinical trials do so during periods of extraordinary clinical fright. They want access to treatment and are not as focused on reading through the informed consent paperwork. And, as many of us in this room may know, having a higher education seems to have little effect regarding comprehension when it comes to informed consent paperwork," said Smith. He added, "We need to increase participation in clinical trials among underrepresented groups," and named several examples of such groups:

- Individuals with impaired health literacy
- Individuals for whom English is not their first language
- Individuals with lower educational attainment
- Individuals from lower socioeconomic backgrounds

INTRODUCTION 3

Smith also highlighted immigrant populations as being especially underrepresented and encouraged the medical community to take the lead on increasing immigrant population participation.

ORGANIZATION OF THE PROCEEDINGS

The remainder of this proceedings summarizes the discussions that took place throughout the workshop and highlights key lessons, practical strategies, and the needs and opportunities for using the principles of health literacy to increase quality and outcomes in clinical trials. Chapter 2 explores the ethical imperative of incorporating health literacy practices in clinical trials. Chapter 3 offers strategies for improving recruitment and retention in clinical trials by embedding health literacy practices along every phase of the trial. Chapter 4 provides several examples of health literacy practices in action, including strategies for implementing interventions, improving patient centeredness, and addressing common barriers to participation in clinical trials. Chapter 5 summarizes a panel discussion on future steps and Chapter 6 covers possible research and policy directions along with reflections from the roundtable members and two workshop speakers. Appendix B contains the speaker biosketches.

2

Health Literacy as an Ethical Imperative in Clinical Trials

The workshop's first session featured two keynote speakers who provided an overview of health literacy as an ethical imperative in clinical trials. Barbara E. Bierer, professor of medicine and faculty co-director of the Multi-Regional Clinical Trials Center of Brigham and Women's Hospital and Harvard (MRCT Center), offered her perspective on why health literacy matters. Deborah Collyar, founder and president of Patient Advocates in Research (PAIR), then discussed how health literacy helps patients make decisions. The two presentations were followed by a discussion with the audience, moderated by Lawrence G. Smith, founding dean of the Donald and Barbara Zucker School of Medicine at Hofstra/Northwell and physician-in-chief at Northwell Health.

WHY HEALTH LITERACY MATTERS

Barbara E. Bierer, Professor of Medicine and Faculty Director, Multi-Regional Clinical Trials Center of Brigham and Women's Hospital and Harvard

Bierer opened her keynote address by noting that her presentation on why health literacy matters in clinical trials represents the work of about 50 people, and she emphasized that she is "only one spokesperson" for the larger group. The MRCT Center, she noted, is a research and policy center that focuses on "conduct, oversight, ethics, and regulatory environment for clinical trials with the purpose of improving [their] integrity, safety, and rigor." The MRCT Center pursues this work with academic credibility and as an independent convener, she added. The MRCT Center facilitates its research and policy efforts by engaging a range of diverse stakeholders involved in clinical research. According to Bierer, those stakeholders include pharmaceutical companies, contract research organizations, academicians, patients, patient advocates, regulatory folks, and others. "We work to create actionable, ethical, and practical solutions," she said, "and the MRCT Center works to deliver practical tools and resources that individuals can use."

Bierer noted that the MRCT Center has been focusing on improving health literacy in clinical trials for about 1.5 years, but that the idea actually started several years before that, when the MRCT Center was focused on returning individual and aggregate summary results to participants. "It's an unmet need," she said, "and participants really would like to get the results of their clinical trials participation and almost never do." The MRCT Center team had analyzed the clinical research pathway, noting multiple opportunities for the implementation of health literacy practices ranging from "access and information in advance of anyone getting sick to the end of the clinical trial when [investigators] communicate [the participants'] individual and summary results."

Health-Literate Practices to Address Disparities and Increase Participant Trust

Bierer set the stage by highlighting that the MRCT Center team hoped to improve the diversity of participants in their trials with health literacy best practices (i.e., sharing information in ways that support understanding and autonomous action). She added, "clinical trials in the U.S. lack appropriate diverse representation and we don't know the role of health literacy in reinforcing that inequity." She added that the ethical foundation of clinical research is voluntary and informed consent: anyone who considers entering and then participating in a clinical trial deserves to understand the trial; its goals, risks, burdens, and potential benefits; and the alternatives to participation. Bierer also identified some of the groups who need to "be around the table" when it comes to developing health-literate practices for clinical trials:

- Funders
- Sponsors
- Investigators and study teams
- Individuals representing the Institutional Review Boards (IRBs)
- Potential clinical trial participants
- Families and caregivers of potential participants

All of these groups could collaborate to create health-literate study materials. Bierer added that such a collaboration could increase trust in the system among participants, their caregivers, and their families. When Bierer began working on the health literacy in clinical research project at the MRCT Center, about 50 people volunteered to participate. Bierer explained that the volunteers adopted a "multidimensional" definition of health literacy:

> This is not only about plain language. This is about numeracy, visualization, navigation, cultural competencies, and developing a system that is health literate.[1] It is about developing actionable tools.

Bierer added that the workshop audience may be more than familiar with the concept that health literacy represents two-sided communication, but it is worth repeating:

> It is not the responsibility of the person receiving information to try and make sense of it; it is clearly the communicator who is responsible for ensuring that the information they communicate is understood by the target audience. The target audience should be in a setting where they are comfortable saying they don't understand and asking to go over information again.

Beyond two groups of individuals communicating, there is also a systems problem, she said. Collectively, "we don't invest in making health-literate communications, training, and education." She added that the workshop audience had a high level of health literacy expertise, which was often not the case for investigators and research personnel. "Why is that?" she asked, adding:

> [Health literacy] is foundational to the ethical conduct of clinical research, and the very foundation of how we approach clinical research is through voluntary informed consent. In the absence of demonstrated understanding, how can you really know that somebody is consenting in an informed and voluntary way?

Bierer noted that equitable access to research is also deeply important. She added that she remained skeptical about the degree to which investigators and their institutions have embraced the health literacy concept, and whether IRBs consider it their responsibility to "provide oversight to health-literate communications." There are also resourcing implications,

---

[1] "Visualization" as referred to in this presentation refers to graphics, images, and clear design strategies to enhance written and verbal content. "Navigation" refers to an individual's ability to move through a given health care/research system or process.

she added, including time, money, and people, all of which need to be invested into the process of implementing health-literate practices in clinical trials. She continued,

> I go beyond the ethics to say that it is also important for the scientific integrity of the trial and the generalizability of the research. If you do not have a diverse participation in the trial, you do not know how generalizable the results of the trial will be. Our trials should reflect the population that will be affected by the disease and likely to benefit from whatever intervention is being studied. Better communication will also enhance compliance and, thus, data validity. If people don't understand what they are supposed to do in a research procedure or for their follow-up care, they can't possibly comply with those expectations—and I would posit that it's also better for retention if somebody really feels that they understand why they are contributing to science and what they may get out of it.

Health Literacy in the Clinical Trial Life Cycle

Bierer said that at the MRCT Center, they think that

> [the clinical trial life cycle] goes from discovery, from access to education, all the way through to the end of the study and communication, and clear communication is essential throughout. But we will go somewhat further. We posit that beyond health literacy, we should strive to ensure clinical trial literacy. People can understand the health implications and still not be comfortable with words, concepts, or underlying clinical trial expectations and assumptions. What does that look like? Building relationships with and developing the general research information for the community of interest, it starts with access in that education and moves toward thoughtful and multiformat study-specific recruitment materials and procedures. I am not talking about written consent. I am talking about the process. I am talking about thinking about informed consent in a different way. We are living in a world with YouTube and other formats and we should be availing ourselves of visual methodologies. I think we should provide detailed study information to support informed decision making, and then provide study participation materials that are appropriate.

Finally, Bierer said, being attentive to health literacy from the beginning supports communication and information sharing at the end of the trial. "You know your target audience by this point," and would be able to communicate appropriately, she said.

> The information you gather from participants throughout the life cycle of the clinical trial should feed into making your next iteration better. Further, this is a two-way, dynamic engagement. Bilateral engagement with the

participants and partnerships with those participants are always of benefit. You learn more from talking to participants or potential participants than you do sitting down with a dictionary.

Existing Tools to Improve Health Literacy in Clinical Trials

Bierer highlighted some of the work the MRCT Center had done that focused on access, education, and developing patient-facing materials and resources.

Participant Brochures

Harvard Catalyst has developed 25 brochures for potential clinical trial participants, in 15 languages, which "are all health literate and all reviewed by IRBs and have gone through health-literate sorts of revisions by [patient advocacy] professionals."[2] She added that, in order to ensure the translated issues would work well, they collaborated with people who were based in the countries in which the brochures would be distributed. Bierer invited the workshop to review the brochures and make suggestions for improvements or for other brochures to be developed.[3]

Plain-Language Dictionaries

She also highlighted an existing plain-language dictionary, which was not developed by the MRCT Center but by UnitedHealth Group.[4] "UnitedHealth Group has done a brilliant job of making a 17,000-word dictionary available—and it's translated into Spanish and Portuguese. There is no need to reinvent the wheel." She added that the MRCT Center has begun to invest in developing a suite of terms that are used almost exclusively in clinical trial contexts to supplement existing efforts. In addition to plain language, Bierer noted that numeracy is "incredibly important," adding, "it's not just visuals that are easy to understand, like a pie chart." She added that it included clarifying the relative risk and absolute risk when talking with a clinical trials participant.

---

[2] For more information about Harvard Catalyst, see https://www.catalyst.harvard.edu (accessed August 6, 2019).

[3] To read more about the process of developing brochures and other educational materials for research participants, see www.cambridge.org/core/services/aop-cambridge-core/content/view/55A05866C8E3EF81181A311D9382FAEC/S205986611800016Xa.pdf/development_of_a_plainlanguage_library_of_educational_resources_for_research_participants.pdf (accessed October 16, 2019).

[4] For more information about UnitedHealth Group's Just Plain Clear® Glossary, see www.justplainclear.com/en (accessed August 6, 2019).

Health-Literate, Patient-Facing, Patient-Centered Materials

Bierer showed the audience several examples of older consent forms, with dense amounts of small text. She pointed to Merck and Health Literacy Media as leaders in the field of developing patient information materials that are clear and useful. She added that she has seen a rising appreciation of patient participation, of how patient engagement can make clinical trials more patient-centric, and of how patient voices in developing clinical trials matter. She continued, "If you work with the community and use their language, by default you are more likely to be health literate in your communications."

Potential Systems Changes to Improve Health Literacy in Clinical Trials

Bierer emphasized that health literacy is a responsibility of the entire system, and it is not up to the communicator or patient alone. She added that there is a need for both corporate and individual commitments to communication and patient engagement throughout the process. "Trials are engineered to deliver results," she said, "and they should be engineered to deliver results that are important to participants, patients, their loved ones, and to society—not because it's the investigator's favorite question."

The process of incorporating health literacy into clinical trials requires dissection, analysis, and reengineering, Bierer said, and that goes beyond simply having plain-language terms, but rather toward their use and meaning in the culture in which they will be used. Bierer suggested that there should be more focus on design, numeracy, visualization, and education and training for all individuals involved in clinical trials. She also named a few factors going forward that would improve the use of health literacy practices in clinical trials:

- A commitment to provide resources required by relevant stakeholders
- Use of tools and resources to decrease the perceived burden of clear communication
- Iterative quality improvement of all materials
- Incentive structures to reward the right behaviors

Regarding the last point, Bierer pointed out that any researchers who start a clinical trial will then add that accomplishment to their curriculum vitae (CV). If a trial is not finished, the participants are put at risk without the possibility of benefit, Bierer said, and the investigator is not prohibited from keeping the clinical trial as an accomplishment on their CV.

Bierer closed her talk with the news that the MRCT Center is developing a website dedicated to health literacy resources for clinical trials, and she invited the workshop audience to collaborate with her team.[5]

HEALTH LITERACY HELPS PATIENTS MAKE DECISIONS: A PATIENT PERSPECTIVE[6]

*Deborah Collyar, Founder and President,
Patient Advocates in Research*

Collyar opened her keynote by offering a "real-world approach" from a patient perspective on what it is like to be involved in clinical trials. Collyar noted that she hoped the workshop would present opportunities to accelerate the availability of information to people at the time they need it, throughout diagnosis, treatments, and clinical trial considerations, and with clinical trial results summaries.

In the "U.S. disease crisis system," Collyar said, explaining that she thinks the term is more appropriate than "health care system," each individual is relabeled as a "patient" as soon as they are diagnosed with a medical condition or illness, and the more serious it is, the more acute the difference becomes. From a patient perspective, she continued, "it's like being catapulted onto a different planet without a roadmap, dictionary, or any type of survival training. You feel totally alone and ill-equipped for what you're about to hear."

She added that it is important to know that when someone is diagnosed with an illness or disease, their body often puts them into a physiological, traumatic, stress state that causes both physical and emotional symptoms[7]:

> It's the strangest thing to hear sounds, see lips moving, and focus harder than you have ever focused in your life, and information doesn't connect. And it's not because anyone is inept or uneducated. Their body is trying to protect them.

She added that this is why she and her colleagues always tell people to bring another person with them or record their conversation, so they can listen to it alone or with loved ones later and try to process the information. "The more we can help [patients] in that situation, the better," she said,

---

[5] See https://mrctcenter.org/health-literacy (accessed October 21, 2019).

[6] This section is based on the presentation by Deborah Collyar, and her statements are not endorsed or verified by the National Academies of Sciences, Engineering, and Medicine.

[7] See www.medlineplus.gov/stress.html (accessed October 16, 2019), www.apa.org/helpcenter/stress-body (accessed October 16, 2019), and https://store.samhsa.gov/system/files/sma13-4775.pdf (accessed October 16, 2019) for more information about traumatic stress.

"and the more we can help health care providers in that situation, the better." She added that this would *not* include distributing medical literature to patients, because it is not helpful—even when the shock wears off, there are too many terms that people do not understand.

Another point that is very important, Collyar continued, is that when someone is finally diagnosed with their final illness or condition, "they have probably gone through many different medical providers and many subspecialties, and may have received diagnoses that were not correct. They may even have been treated for an illness or a condition they did not have. That happens too often." There are plenty of ways to breed mistrust among oncology patients, she continued. Collyar emphasized that she believes there are myriad opportunities to engage and inform patients about clinical research and clinical trials throughout their diagnosis and treatment experience. But common problems that add to the mistrust of the medical community include medical professionals that

- misdiagnose patients,
- treat patients as data repositories,
- fail to consider what is in it for the patient, and
- fail to consider the significant costs for patients and their families.

She elaborated on her last point regarding costs:

Of course, we talk about the cost of drugs now, which are astronomical and totally out of reach for a lot of people. A lot of people ask me a question I have a very hard time answering: "Why would I want to support research when all they do is produce drugs nobody can afford?"

We need to talk about that more openly. There are many costs for a patient. There is a cost to their family; there is a cost to their work situation; there is a cost to their social situation. Sometimes, there is a stigma involved [with a medical diagnosis or treatment]. These costs affect a person's ability to manage their illness or disease, and their medical visits.

Collyar noted that she has heard of patients being "blamed" for a lack of interest in clinical trials because only 3–5 percent of patients enroll in clinical trials, but studies show that people *are* interested in clinical research (Anderson et al., 2018; *Applied Clinical Trials*, 2007; DasMahapatra et al., 2017). Patients are often willing to consider clinical trials as part of their treatment decision-making process, but "very few of them actually go to a doctor who does clinical trials. That's a large part of the problem."

The other part of the problem with clinical trial enrollment and retention, Collyar added, is both the limited participant eligibility for clinical trials, and the number of patients interested in participating compared with the clinical trials that currently exist: there is not a clinical trial to suit the needs of every single patient. If we truly mean to engage and center patients, she said, then "we actually have to start thinking differently about the way we conduct clinical research."

Words Matter

Collyar emphasized how overwhelming medical information after a diagnosis can be. She noted that while experiencing shock from a serious diagnosis, patients are often also exposed to unfamiliar medical terms and concepts in a short period of time. This common occurrence, Collyar explained, prompted her to develop material for PAIR called "Words Matter," which highlights terms that are commonly used but may have different meanings outside of clinical settings (see Table 2-1). She asked the audience to consider whether a "negative test" result would be considered good or bad from the patient's perspective. "If you take a pregnancy test, and you want to get pregnant, is [a negative test] good or bad? If you don't want to get pregnant, is [a negative test] good or bad? We have to think about that." Collyar added that there are several terms commonly used in medical settings that do not always mean what patients think they do. "We need to stop saying 'cure' until it *does* mean 'oh, good, I'm never going to have to worry about this disease again.'"

TABLE 2-1 Words Matter: Differences in Medical/Scientific Terms Among Medical Professionals Compared with the General Public

Term	Scientific/Medical Definition	Public Understanding
Negative test	"That's too bad."	"This is good, right?"
Positive test	"That's too bad."	"This is good, right?"
Cure	"5-year survival rate"	"Never again"
Tumor mutation burden	"Good!"	"Sounds bad…?"
Support services	"Help science"	"Fit a medical condition into my life"
Lay	"All nonscientists"	"[Lie] down?"
Environment	"Patient-controlled"	"External forces"
Community	"Nonacademic center"	"Where I live"
Medical advance	"Incremental adjustment"	"A cure"

SOURCE: Adapted from a presentation by Deborah Collyar at the workshop Health Literacy in Clinical Trials: Practice and Impact on April 11, 2019.

"Patients want better treatment, not just more treatment," said Collyar. Part of better treatment is having answers and plans tailored specifically for them, not just other patients, she added. For example, she said:

> Metastatic cancer patients want treatment that will work for them. They don't want to be used as a surrogate for earlier-stage patients anymore. They have their own needs and issues that must be addressed—and they rarely are in clinical trials.

Another promising area of treatment is immunotherapies for cancer patients. There is great promise in immunotherapies, Collyar said, but only a minority of cancer patients are helped by them. "We need to set expectations correctly and properly for everyone so we don't oversell or overhype it. A lot of tumors don't respond to immunotherapy." It can be a layer of treatment for cancer patients, she continued, but patients also need realistic expectations. For example, she said, fewer patients experience adverse side effects or adverse events (AEs) from immunotherapy than from chemotherapy (Baxi et al., 2018; Marshall et al., 2018; Puzanov et al., 2017). However, she continued, when patients do experience immunotherapy AEs, "they are horrible."

Duration of response is another concept that can confuse patients and participants in clinical trials. "When someone hears that they have had a complete response from their cancer treatment, they think they are done. They don't know it's defined as a 3-month or 6-month period in the clinical trial. We have to do a better job of explaining what those terms actually mean."

Collyar noted that she served as co-chair on the Cancer and Leukemia Group B's Committee on Advocacy, Research Communications, Ethics, and Disparities (CARE) from 1998 through 2010, and helped them create better clinical trials with better results, especially for patients. "Feasibility is a big part," she added. As patient advocates, "we not only help with that, we also help sponsors understand how to identify and solve some of the issues that patients have, not just for the scientific compound itself." Collyar has also been involved in developing recruitment plans with regulators and IRBs, helping explain to patient communities what clinical research is and why they might want to consider it. CARE was one of the first groups that advocated for providing participants in clinical trials with their results, doing so in the late 1990s. To emphasize the point that clinical trials need to center on the patient's perspective, she asked the workshop to say which of the following two statements should be used:

- The patient failed the treatment.
- The treatment failed the patient.

She urged the workshop to avoid using the first option, to avoid blaming patients for the failure of a treatment. "This is more than a semantic exercise," Collyar emphasized. She added, "We have to rethink the way that we approach medicine and clinical trials if we want to make an impact on how patients feel about them."

What Patients Want to Know About Clinical Trials

Collyar pointed out that a primary concern for patients is about the feeling of total isolation, postdiagnosis. Medical professionals can help patients understand that they are not alone, that there are others who share their diagnosis, and that there is precedent for participating in clinical research and even what the results of that research have been thus far. Collyar added that clinical researchers and medical professionals should constantly consider questions a patient might ask or help them consider those questions because "ongoing communication is key" (see Box 2-1 for sample questions).

Patients also want to hear about the results of the study they participated in and contributed to. On the topic of plain-language summaries, Collyar expressed excitement about a relatively new regulation from the European Medicines Agency (EMA) that requires the results of each clinical trial carried out in the European Union (EU) to be made publicly available.[8] Though

---

BOX 2-1
Possible Patient Questions Regarding Clinical Trials

Collyar advised that clinical researchers keep the following questions in mind when engaging with patients and clinical research participants:

- What are we doing in the trial?
- Why are we doing the trial?
- What should I expect during the trial?
- Is there a safe word to exit the trial? What is it?
- What would happen to me if I withdraw from the trial?
- What is going to happen to me after the trial is over?

SOURCE: Adapted from a presentation by Deborah Collyar at the workshop Health Literacy in Clinical Trials: Practice and Impact on April 11, 2019.

---

[8] Clinical Trial Regulation EU No. 536/2014 requires consistent rules for conducting clinical trials throughout the EU and that information on the authorization, conduct, and results of each trial be made publicly available. For more information on the regulation, see https://www.ema.europa.eu/en/human-regulatory/research-development/clinical-trials/clinical-trial-regulation (accessed August 29, 2019).

the EMA also uses the term "lay summaries," Collyar noted that she prefers "plain-language summaries," because none of the definitions of "lay" identify it as being nonmedical, and several of them are derogatory. She continued, "there is no reason we can't call it a public trial result summary," adding that the plain-language element of the summaries is just one part of health literacy. Collyar explained that plain-language summaries represent an opportunity to influence the field and improve the patient experience at large.

Another important concept to consider is the option to switch treatments (also called a crossover) in a clinical trial, Collyar said. This is an important consideration because if a patient is assigned to one arm of a randomized study and their cancer comes back, they could switch to the other arm of the study, ideally without jeopardizing the generalizability or statistical significance of its results. Collyar added that a white paper was published in 2016 describing how to report results in trials that involved treatment switching (Green Park Collaborative, 2016).

What Clinical Trials Should Really Be About

Collyar said crossover designs are just one example of clinical researchers rethinking clinical trial design. She added that the trials should be designed and conducted with clinical use in mind, considering "how patients would actually use this drug." Although patient-reported outcomes (PROs) started as a means of reporting AEs, Collyar said, they encompass much more than that and should be utilized to reflect more of the patient's experience in the trial. Collyar added that the U.S. Food and Drug Administration (FDA) and other regulatory agencies have been very receptive to using PROs in the approval process.

Collyar observed that, because of shorter FDA approval cycles for clinical research, there are many more questions left unanswered. Collyar urged clinical researchers to focus on finding ways to answer those questions, even after drugs are commercially available. Lingering questions include the following:

- What are the long-term effects of the drug?
- What kind of regimens are best for the drug?
- Which populations does the drug work in?
- Which subtypes of disease benefit the most from the drug?

Collyar added that patients should also be informed about risk evaluation and mitigation strategies (REMS), and how they can allow drugs to have shorter approval cycles, while reducing the risk of AEs.[9]

---

[9] FDA can require drug manufacturers to develop REMS for certain medications with serious safety concerns to help ensure the benefits of the medication outweigh its risks. For more information about REMS, see https://www.fda.gov/drugs/drug-safety-and-availability/risk-evaluation-and-mitigation-strategies-rems (accessed August 29, 2019).

Closing her presentation, Collyar asked the workshop to remember what patients, clinical research participants, and health care providers need as four Cs: clear communication of content and context.

DISCUSSION

Including Primary Care Providers

Smith opened the panel discussion by noting that, in his experience as a primary care physician (PCP), PCPs are often shut out of their patients' entire clinical trial process. He explained that patients had booked appointments to treat symptoms that were actually AEs from a trial, but as their PCP, he was unaware the patients were enrolled in trials at all. At best, this can cause confusion within a PCP's office, and, at worst, it causes medical complications or mistreatment. He wondered why there were not handouts given to trial participants to share with their PCPs and how to encourage specialists who enroll participants to communicate with PCPs about their patients participating in clinical trials.

Bierer replied that she thought this was a great point, and part of a prior MRCT Center return-of-results project (in which she and Collyar were involved) addressed the disconnect between investigator and health care provider. She noted that early and constant communication to the provider is important, with the participant's consent, especially because trial results take significant time to become available. Because of this, investigators can have trouble identifying and contacting the participants after the study, she added, at a time when many participants have returned to the care of their PCP. And if investigators cannot contact their participants with results, there is only a slim chance they will be able to contact the participants' PCP unless communication had already been established. Improving multiparty communication deserves "significant study, dissection, analysis, and the establishment of whether there are tools we can make available now," she said.

Bierer noted that some trials are now conducted in communities with PCPs as investigators. On the one hand, this keeps PCPs connected to their patients' experiences; on the other hand, it raises a set of ethical issues. However, Bierer said, "we need a system where there is both communication and knowledge."

Collyar agreed and added that most patients want their doctor to know that they are participating in a clinical trial, and most want to continue to see the PCP they have built a relationship with over a course of years. She noted, "We have to make sure that information is available in both directions."

Engaging Stakeholders During Clinical Research

Terry C. Davis from the Louisiana State University Health Sciences Center in Shreveport asked the panelists about their takeaways regarding stakeholder engagement. As the co-chair of a stakeholder engagement group on a particular clinical research project, she asked, "what is the best way to involve stakeholders, and how often?"

Collyar noted that investigators seem to think about "the patient" as a single person, when in fact "there is an entire spectrum, of ages, experiences, cultures, and issues" among patients. "My dream," she added, "is that we actually are able to use clinical trial results in a way that makes our new trials better (including adaptive clinical trial design), so that we're raising the bar on better designs and helping to build better results and impacts for patient communities as new drugs are developed."

Bierer added that not enough is known about stakeholder engagement, particularly in trial design. She noted a few questions she thought should be answered:

- How many patients should be consulted on trial design?
- How many focus groups would you need to conduct?
- Is the focus group diverse enough?

She added that materials are often reviewed by trial participants but only initially, and then the iterative process stops, although she believes it could be continually improved and tailored.

Education and the Informed Consent Process

Michael McKee from the University of Michigan Medical School noted that the deaf and hard-of-hearing communities and, more broadly, people with disabilities, are all at a disadvantage with regard to accessing information available to the mainstream population. Accordingly, he posed two questions to the panelists:

1. Could you highlight or provide some examples of what has worked in your communities on the educational part before you delve into the consent process?
2. Could you share some examples of different methods of informed consent education—audio, visual, written—that have worked and which approaches might be ideal to use?

Bierer responded first by noting that her experience in this area was anecdotal and not endorsed by any employer or university. If you are asking how to do informed consent well, she said, it is important to appreciate that developing informed consent documents is a serious process. She added that participants may understand one part of an informed consent document initially, and, as the trial proceeds or their participation proceeds, they may recognize the significance of another part of it. As an investigator, she said, "I see it as an ongoing responsibility" to maintain open communication with any participant, to allow any question to be raised at any time in the trial. One important part of the initial informed consent process, for Bierer, is annotating the original document, pulling out what needs to be said, what needs to be asked about the end of each paragraph, and thinking through, in advance, what reflections a participant would need to give in a "teach-back" setting to document comprehension. Once that information is collected, investigators can develop a script to engage with participants about the subject.

Bierer noted that a principle oversight responsibility of IRBs is to monitor and review consent processes, conversations, and documents, although she has seen few consent interactions actually monitored by an IRB professional. She also noted that McKee's question brought up the broader issue of the inclusion of marginalized communities in clinical research. Some of those groups that tend to be excluded are people with disabilities, she said, as well as rural communities and Native American communities.

> We don't do a good job of including them. We don't even know what their issues are ... we should move from a stance of protectionism, which is how we have engaged with vulnerable populations, toward one of inclusion, where we really try and understand what the safety, efficacy, and effectiveness profile of our interventions are, not just drugs and devices, but all interventions for all of the people we serve.

Bierer added that cultural competence should be prioritized among researchers, including having adequate translation and interpretation services, and developing culturally appropriate educational materials.

Collyar noted that therapeutic misconception is also a hurdle when it comes to informed consent. Patients do not see the informed consent process in the same way the research community does, she said, and patients do not necessarily understand the difference between participating in a clinical trial and choosing a treatment that is already available. She also noted that the way this issue has been approached has been unsuccessful—the "misconception" is actually in the research world, because, for the patient, it is actually their treatment.

Patient Safety and Health Literacy in Clinical Trials

Jay Duhig from AbbVie Inc. asked how to help people understand the difference between research and treatment. He cited an issue among some trial participants: clinical research documents instruct participants to tell their study doctor if they experience a certain side effect. Duhig explained that no matter how "health literate" the material is those participants understand that if they report that specific side effect, their treatment will be discontinued. In some cases, participants believe that their treatment from the trial is their best chance for managing their disease, which means that they will not always report a serious side effect if they think it means they will lose the treatment altogether. Duhig continued, "how do we address that from a patient standpoint?"

Addressing therapeutic misconception is a major issue, Collyar agreed. She hears frequently that patients go to their study doctors and "put their best foot forward," describing certain symptoms or side effects they might be experiencing. She added that this is another important reason for having a trusted family member or friend accompany the patient to doctor visits, because they can help create a clearer picture for the study team.

Collyar admitted she was unsure about how to solve the issue, but emphasized that clear communication and expectations were paramount, because patients' understanding that their safety is the highest priority can help frame the way they think about clinical research. She also reiterated how PROs become more important to help resolve these kinds of issues.

Bierer agreed with Collyar and said she thinks setting expectations with participants is often difficult. She wondered if exploring anonymous reporting in a different way might be useful, adding that some patients already use social media in ways that affect their inclusion, exclusion, and/or retention in trials.

The Role of Support Groups in Patient Decision Making

Linda Harris from the U.S. Department of Health and Human Services' Office of Disease Prevention and Health Promotion posed the final question of the panel. "I wanted you to talk about the role of support groups in helping patients make decisions about their clinical trial experience," she said. "Are they friends of those of us who are advocates of health literacy? Could they be recruited to be more helpful?"

Collyar said she thought they could be useful and certainly could be recruited to be more helpful. She noted that the AIDS movement in the early 1990s taught many patients to organize and become activists for their own health. While companies may not allow support groups because of potential bias, Collyar said, patients are talking anyway. "Why not have some control over the discussion that is already there to make sure it's accurate and useful and constructive?" She added that it could debunk some of the urban legends, like "don't tell your doctor about your side effects or you'll be taken off treatment." Collyar said, "That's real in the patient world; many think that."

REFERENCES

Anderson, A., D. Borfitz, and K. Getz. 2018. Global public attitudes about clinical research and patient experiences with clinical trials. *JAMA Network Open* 1(6):e182969. doi: 10.1001/jamanetworkopen.2018.2969.

Applied Clinical Trials. 2007. A survey of survivors: To improve enrollment in oncology trials, one patient advocate group went straight to the source. *Applied Clinical Trials,* July 1, 2007. http://www.appliedclinicaltrialsonline.com/survey-survivors (accessed October 17, 2019).

Baxi, S., A. Yang, R. L. Gennarelli, N. Khan, Z. Wang, L. Boyce, and D. Korenstein. 2018. Immune-related adverse events for anti-PD-1 and anti-PD-L1 drugs: Systematic review and meta-analysis. *BMJ* 360:k793. https://doi.org/10.1136/bmj.k793.

DasMahapatra, P., P. Raja, J. Gilbert, and P. Wicks. 2017. Clinical trials from the patient perspective: Survey in an online patient community. *BMC Health Serv Res* 17(1):166. https://doi.org/10.1186/s12913-017-2090-x.

Green Park Collaborative. 2016. *Best practices for the design, implementation, analysis, and reporting of oncology trials with high rates of treatment switching.* http://www.cmtpnet.org/docs/resources/Treatment_Switching_Guidance_Document_OCT_2016.pdf (accessed August 29, 2019).

Marshall, J., T. Bekaii-Saab, and L. Saltz. 2018. *Immunotherapy hype and oncologists' fear of failure drive "hail Mary" treatments.* https://www.medscape.com/viewarticle/897946 (accessed August 29, 2019).

Puzanov, I., A. Diab, K. Abdallah, C. O. Bingham, 3rd, C. Brogdon, R. Dadu, L. Hamad, S. Kim, M. E. Lacouture, N. R. LeBoeuf, D. Lenihan, C. Onofrei, V. Shannon, R. Sharma, A. W. Silk, D. Skondra, M. E. Suarez-Almazor, Y. Wang, K. Wiley, H. L. Kaufman, and M. S. Ernstoff. 2017. Managing toxicities associated with immune checkpoint inhibitors: Consensus recommendations from the Society for Immunotherapy of Cancer (SITC) Toxicity Management Working Group. *Journal for ImmunoTherapy of Cancer* 5(1):95. doi: 10.1186/s40425-017-0300-z.

3

Embedding Health Literacy in Clinical Trials to Improve Recruitment and Retention

A discussion panel explored how to embed health literacy into clinical trials from the beginning of the process in order to improve recruitment and retention. Annlouise R. Assaf from Pfizer Worldwide Medical and Safety served as the moderator. The panelists included Ebony Boulware, professor of medicine, chief of the Division of General Internal Medicine in the Department of Medicine, vice dean for translational science, and associate vice chancellor for translational research in the School of Medicine at Duke University; Catina O'Leary, president and chief executive officer of Health Literacy Media (HLM); Alicia Staley, senior director, patient engagement for mHealth at Medidata Solutions; and Christopher R. Trudeau, associate professor of medical humanities, University of Arkansas for Medical Sciences, and associate professor of law, Bowen School of Law, University of Arkansas at Little Rock.

Assaf introduced this panel's topics: communicating about clinical trials and preparing for informed consent; health-literate recruitment strategies; and developing health-literate materials. She explained that the panel would discuss what goes into creating health-literate materials and how these efforts go beyond plain language. She also mentioned that the panel would touch on informed consent documents and issues faced by Institutional Review Boards (IRBs); how to enroll minorities with variable health literacy into clinical trials; and the regulatory trend toward health literacy in clinical trials. Each panelist introduced their work and their interests as they related to improving recruitment and retention in clinical trials. Assaf posed several of her own questions for each panelist to discuss, and she then facilitated a discussion between the panelists and the audience. A summary of key points made by each speaker can be found in Box 3-1.

ENROLLING MINORITIES WITH VARIABLE LITERACY IN CLINICAL TRIALS

Ebony Boulware, Professor of Medicine, Chief of the Division of General Internal Medicine in the Department of Medicine, Vice Dean for Translational Science, and Associate Vice Chancellor for Translational Research in the School of Medicine, Duke University

Boulware explained that she and her colleagues have focused on clinical trials that enrolled minorities with various literacy levels. She and her team had mainly worked on behavioral and educational interventions that were implemented in clinical settings, she said, as opposed to drug trials. Boulware noted that, as Bierer had previously alluded to, there is a well-justified history of mistrust regarding the research enterprise on the part of minority populations, specifically the African American population, in

---

BOX 3-1
Key Points Raised by Individual Panelists

- Collaboration with Institutional Review Boards is not only possible but can also be very useful in developing health-literate materials for trial participants. (Boulware, O'Leary)
- To improve participant and patient engagement and/or retention, follow-up calls and home visits are essential. (Boulware, O'Leary, Staley)
- There is a need for more research on optimal ways for trial participants to receive information. (Trudeau)
- User testing and focus group testing should be standard practice in designing trials. (O'Leary, Trudeau)
- Recent regulatory changes in both the United States and the European Union support health-literate practices in clinical trials. (Trudeau)
- It is important to start building relationships with communities of potential participants before the recruitment process starts. (Boulware, Staley)
- Flexibility and collaboration with potential participant communities are keys to successful recruitment and enrollment. (Boulware, O'Leary, Staley)
- Informed consent is a memorialization of the educational process, not a transactional document to be signed. (Trudeau)

SOURCE: Adapted from a panel discussion among Annlouise R. Assaf, Ebony Boulware, Catina O'Leary, Alicia Staley, and Christopher R. Trudeau at the workshop Health Literacy in Clinical Trials: Practice and Impact on April 11, 2019.

the United States.[1] For Boulware that has meant that understanding and identifying with those historically marginalized or mistreated populations in the clinical trials context was a crucial aspect of designing a trial, enrolling participants, and conducting the trial with health literacy competencies. Highlighting three studies in which she and her colleagues had worked on enrolling African American participants, she observed, "We're talking about how we engage people and how we relate to them as real people with real histories."

PREPARED Study—Baltimore, Maryland

The first study Boulware described had enrolled African American patients with kidney failure and who were being treated at dialysis units in Baltimore, Maryland. Participants were randomly assigned to receive either their usual care alone or that care plus culturally tailored educational interventions to improve their shared and informed decision making about their kidney treatments. The enrollment rate was 66 percent, and the retention rate was 80 percent (Boulware et al., 2018).

ACT Study—Baltimore, Maryland

The second study Boulware described focused on African Americans with uncontrolled hypertension, who were being seen in primary care settings. The interventions included a community health worker, blood pressure cuffs, and other educational interventions to improve blood pressure self-management and control. The enrollment rate was 60 percent, and the retention rate was 83 percent (Boulware et al., 2020).

TALKS Study—Durham, North Carolina

The third study was also focused on providing educational and behavioral interventions, as well as financial support intervention, for African American participants at a transplant center in Durham, North Carolina. The study explored whether the interventions helped participants when considering a kidney transplant. The enrollment rate was 65 percent, and the retention rate was 87 percent (Strigo et al., 2015).

---

[1] For more information regarding minority population mistrust in the clinical research enterprise, see http://buildingtrustumd.org/unit/informed-decision-making/learning-from-the-past (accessed October 17, 2019).

LESSONS LEARNED FROM BEHAVIORAL TRIALS OF AFRICAN AMERICANS

Boulware observed that the activities were fairly diverse, but the numbers for recruitment and retention were "reasonably successful," because patient and participant engagement before, during, and throughout the studies had been a critical component of their trial designs (see Table 3-1 for complete statistics on the studies). She added that there were several approaches to these studies that improved the enrollment and retention of diverse populations with various literacy levels, and that investigators should do the following:

- Engage potential participant populations well before the study starts
- Be willing to substantially change designs or materials from the original protocol to accommodate what the potential participant population thinks is more appropriate
- Work with IRBs to clarify and tailor consent forms and communicate with potential participants more clearly
- Tailor recruitment letters, not just with plain language but with accessible and clear formatting, straightforward messaging, and cultural sensitivity
- Continue to tailor materials throughout the study
- Follow up via phone calls and home visits, in addition to the usual postcards or letters, to keep participants engaged and to help them understand the importance of their involvement

Boulware added that she was excited by other examples of newer consent forms she had seen earlier in the day, as well the use of video and graphics to engage and educate potential participants. She asked the workshop to consider whether retention and enrollment are the best metrics of success for a trial, and whether investigators should consider other factors:

> Should we really be thinking about other metrics that have to do with the experience of the participant and their satisfaction with their engagement with the trial itself that goes above and beyond the receipt of the intervention?

TABLE 3-1 Three Small Clinical Trials with African American Participants

Study	Final N	Enrollment Numbers	Enrollment Rate	Retention Rate	Retention Rate by Arm
PREPARED	92	Screened/eligible: 189 Declined: 54 Consented: 105	66%	80%	Arm 1: 84% Arm 2: 73% Arm 3: 84%
ACT	159	Screened/eligible: 308 Declined: 93 Consented: 185	60%	83%	Arm 1: 84% Arm 2: 73% Arm 3: 84%
TALKS	300	Screened/eligible: 465 Declined: 106 Excluded for other reason: 147 Consented: 300	65%	87%	Arm 1: 89% Arm 2: 86% Arm 3: 87%

SOURCES: Adapted from a presentation by Ebony Boulware at the workshop Health Literacy in Clinical Trials: Practice and Impact on April 11, 2019; Boulware et al., 2018, 2020; Strigo et al., 2015.

HEALTH-LITERATE MATERIALS FOR RECRUITMENT AND RETENTION

Catina O'Leary, President and Chief Executive Officer, Health Literacy Media

O'Leary emphasized that it is important to think of health-literate materials beyond consent forms and plain-language summaries. She noted that recruitment for clinical trials can involve a range of materials: flyers, letters, social media messaging, websites, and press releases (see Figure 3-1). These materials can be utilized in print or multimedia formats, she added, and "every single material developed to communicate with people about the possible study can benefit from health-literate, usable, accessible language."

O'Leary pointed out that printed materials about studies can be underutilized by clinical trial investigators and participants:

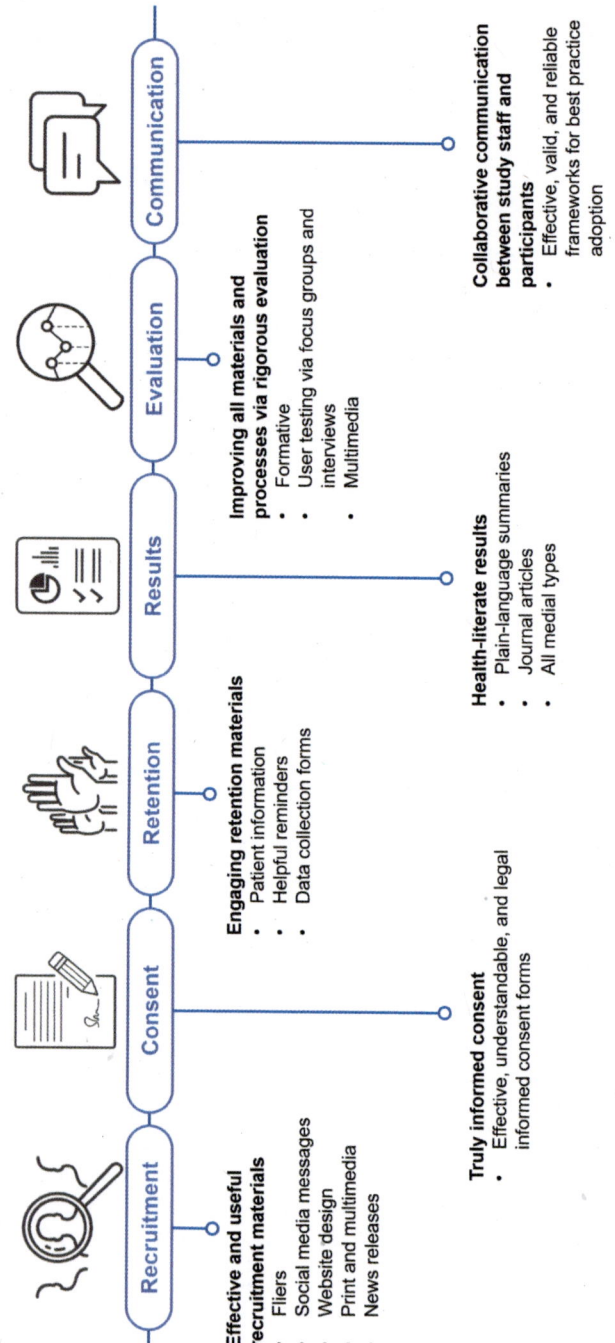

FIGURE 3-1 Health literacy through the clinical trials process.
SOURCE: Adapted from a presentation by Catina O'Leary at the workshop Health Literacy in Clinical Trials: Practice and Impact on April 11, 2019.

> People depend on verbal communication to help [hearing] people understand processes. We know that doesn't work well all the time. People need to be able to go home and review study information, and talk it through with people around them.

She added that there are plenty of ways to engage participants during and after trials, noting that journal articles about the trials should not only be accessible but usable and understandable. Each process within a trial should be rigorously evaluated, she said, but also usable by participants and others. She shared three examples of print materials that HLM had adapted to include health-literate practices.

Sample Informed Consent Form

O'Leary shared two versions of the same sample consent form: one before the health literacy adaptations, and one after. Janssen's investigators spent a lot of time looking at what participants would need for a global consent form, she said. She added that they performed a lot of user testing, and co-designed the material with users. She noted that one might not expect users to care much about the details of consent form design, but every person in the focus groups cared about the colors, words, and even how heavy the lines were between the sections, or how visually demarcated different segments of the trials were. O'Leary said that each of those elements helped users "understand the difference between what happens when participants are screened, when participants are in the treatment period, and when investigators perform follow-up after the trial."

The timelines "really mattered" to users, O'Leary continued. When the forms used colors to separate blocks within the timeline, it made more sense to the users, and they really appreciated that. She also noted that HLM converted original paragraphs of text into a table, underscoring how helpful the visual elements were for users. Adding that the updated informed consent form was "not controversial," she emphasized that IRBs are accustomed to reviewing tables instead of text so developing consent forms like HLM's could make more patients and participants happy without impeding approval. "I would recommend having conversations [with other investigators] about using forms like this," she said.

Sample Participant Study Guide

O'Leary showed another example of an original participant study guide alongside a newer version, adapted by HLM for Merck. The original, she noted, is dense with text, titled "Injection Guide for Study Drug or Placebo—Panel A, Days 1–5, and Panel B, Days 6–10," while the adapted guide is a more visual and colorful guide, titled "How to give yourself the study medicine." She continued:

> There are a lot of pieces about this guide that just jump out—the use of color, the boxes to chunk information, headings that really make a lot of sense for people. But the most dramatic piece of this is the image at the bottom of the drawings. An artist drew what it looks like to take the injection and how people should use it. This drawing tests really well, and people understand what this means and how to hold the medicine and how to give themselves the medicine. They have both the visual image and the words to go along with it.
>
> The drawings are quite simple, culturally, as well. By using drawings instead of images, the guide doesn't make any assumptions about who you are or what it means to be using it.

Sample Trial Results Summary

O'Leary's third and final example was a clinical trial summary. In the original summary, the text is dense and full of jargon, she noted. There were several components to adapting the summary to make it health literate. She explained that the first page has a short summary of everything that happened in the trial. "What we know from patients," O'Leary said, is that patients are "quite happy to read 8 or 10 pages of your summary after they know if a trial has happened with people like them, and whether it made a difference. In that case, they really want to dig in, but they don't want to do it until they are certain it applies to them. They don't want to expend the mental energy."

Because of this, she said, HLM put that information into an executive-level summary, using color chunks, clear headings, and bold titles with clear information. The adapted summary "gets all the elements that are important for participant safety but utilizes a couple of sentences that seem to work well for people," she said. O'Leary added, "We test these and patients really understand it."

O'Leary described the story of a 35-year-old study participant who benefited from the health-literate trial summaries. He had a chronic condition that left him with pain and physical disfigurement—so severe that he dropped out of school, she said, and he had been frequently misdiagnosed.

> It took a long time to get reasonable treatment. But he said that when he read the [HLM] summary, he understood his condition for the first time and knew what was going on with his body. After participating in trials for many years, after his whole life being affected, it took a summary that was well-written to explain what was going on. And because of that, he

said, he felt hopeful: that understanding led to hope and I think that's really important.

TECHNOLOGICAL TOOLS TO IMPROVE PATIENT EXPERIENCES

Alicia Staley, Senior Director of Patient Engagement, mHealth Solutions, Medidata

Staley opened by quoting Dr. Warner Slack, an electronic health record pioneer who argued that "patients are the most underutilized resource in healthcare."[2] She noted that her personal patient experience shaped much of the work she did at Medidata. Staley is a three-time cancer survivor, and in 2011, she co-founded the #bcsmcancercommunity social media community. The online community fosters information sharing among breast cancer patients, she said.

Regarding patient comprehension and understanding, Staley explained that she referred to it as the "Charlie Brown theory of clinical trial comprehension," because adults and teachers in the Charlie Brown cartoon only ever communicate by making the sounds of a muted trombone. When you are first diagnosed with cancer or trying to make a clinical trial, she said, "that's exactly what you hear. Something like 'blah, blah blah, informed consent, blah blah blah, and sign here.'"

As a patient, when you receive lot of information, Staley said, you are often not given the proper context in which to evaluate it, take it in, or process it in a way that really makes sense for you in a critical moment. People learn and process information in different ways, Staley noted. "Some people have to take information in through a book, while others need video or audio. We have to be able to present information in a way patients can receive it." She urged the workshop attendees to consider the context of the patient receiving information:

- Have they just received a new diagnosis?
- Are they returning after one treatment or another has failed?
- What are the technological inputs this patient is encountering?
- Is information being presented over the Web?
- Is information being presented in a clinic or on a tablet?
- How do you judge the comprehension level of the patient?

---

[2] For more information about Dr. Warner Slack and his work, see https://www.bmj.com/content/bmj/362/bmj.k3194.full.pdf (accessed September 17, 2019).

Staley added that she had several doctors over the years ask whether she had understood their conversation. She said her first reaction was always "yes, yes, yes, I've got it," while she walked out of the clinic room, overwhelmed with no context or way to comprehend any of the information she had just received. Now, she said, she knows better:

> I have to leave the appointment, take time to process, and then come back to my doctor and talk about it more. I've been fortunate to be with the same oncology and primary care team now for more than 25 years. They've worked with me to learn how I take in information so they know I might need an extra appointment or a phone call follow-up or an e-mail follow-up to process what they have shared with me. We have to be flexible enough to allow for those kinds of interactions to take place in clinical trials.

Staley urged the workshop attendees to consider "educated consent" as a twin to the informed consent process. "Yes," she said, "there is a [legal] informed consent process where a patient needs to sign off on their participation, but what can we do to infuse education around that process?" She believes, she said, that investigators do not focus enough on education in this context, which is a true multimodal learning opportunity. "We have to build multimodal learning opportunities into the whole consent process. Are you an auditory learner? Are you a visual learner? Do you need to step away from the information for a moment and process it over time?"

Staley reiterated the importance of communicating and presenting information to caregiving teams who support patients. Patients often rely on family and friends to help them through the diagnosis and treatment process, she added. "Are we doing enough so that the patient can confidently go back to their family or care team to share updates or solicit input?" She highlighted something she had heard Collyar say earlier in the day: "The right information at the right time in the right context is really the key for truly engaging patients in clinical research."

Staley summarized by emphasizing three components of best practices for technology improving patient experiences in clinical trials:

- Design: Are you creating material with the patient perspective in mind?
- Engagement: Are you building engagement points for the patient to continually learn throughout the process? What works best—audio, video, interactive applications, paper?
- Activation: What's the environment for information sharing? Can the patient actually act on the information you are presenting to them? Are numbers—figures or statistics—useful information the patient would know what to do with?

REGULATORY CHANGES IN CLINICAL TRIALS

Christopher R. Trudeau, Associate Professor of Medical Humanities, University of Arkansas for Medical Sciences, and Associate Professor of Law, Bowen School of Law, University of Arkansas at Little Rock

Regulations Informing Health Literacy Practices in Clinical Research

Trudeau explained that he viewed his role as an amplifier of the previous panelists. The regulatory context supports all of the activities and examples the other speakers had shared, he said. There are three recent regulatory changes that promote integrating health literacy into clinical trials: two among the European Union (EU) and one in the United States:

- An EU regulation about clinical trials lay summaries
- The EU General Data Protection Regulation (GDPR)
- The U.S. Common Rule revisions

Referring to the controversy over the term "lay summaries," Trudeau noted that everyone could be a "lay" person, depending on the context. "You might be a Ph.D. in epidemiology but you're a lay person in the law to me." The European Union now requires lay- or plain-language summaries, accessible to participants of clinical trials, as Collyar had mentioned during her presentation. The GDPR, Trudeau explained, is a regulation that protects the data of those living in the European Union.[3] When seeking consent, he continued, organizations should ensure that they use clear and plain language in all cases. This means, he added, the message should be easily understandable for the average person and not only for lawyers. He noted that the language of the GDPR also recognizes that minors merit specific protection when it comes to data protection, and the GDPR requires that any communication addressed to children be written in plain language so they can easily understand. It is a broad regulation, Trudeau said, but it has "huge implications" for multinational clinical trials because it applies to any type of data collected from anyone while in the European Union.

---

[3] One section of the GDPR focuses on strengthening the conditions for user consent, forbidding the use of illegible terms, and conditions full of legalese. "The request for consent must be given in an intelligible and easily accessible form, with the purpose for data processing attached to that consent. Consent must be clear and distinguishable from other matters and provided in an intelligible and easily accessible form, using clear and plain language. It must be as easy to withdraw consent as it is to give it" (Trunomi and CommVault, 2018).

The U.S. Common Rule revisions "really support what it is we're trying to do here today," Trudeau said. Having taken complete effect in January 2019, it is the "regulatory hammer that we can use to help encourage others and actually promote health literacy throughout not only the consent process but the entire clinical trial process as well," he added.

The Common Rule revision requires that research consent materials be understandable, Trudeau continued, quoting from the *Federal Register*:

> [It] must be organized and presented in a way that does not merely provide lists of isolated facts, but rather facilitates the prospective subject's or legally authorized representative's understanding of the reason why one might or might not want to participate. (GPO, 2017)

Referring back to the original and revised informed consent documents that O'Leary had shared previously, he lauded Janssen for embracing the challenge to facilitate participant understandings of the timeline, the different stages of the trials, and what happens with each trial visit. "So if you are at an organization where your IRB is not quite up to speed or your organization itself is not, you now have some regulatory support" for incorporating health literacy into your trials, Trudeau said. The change requiring that consent needs to begin with key information, said Trudeau, is "great for us in the health literacy world because it recognizes the individuality of consent, whereas the templates that cover every study, from low risk to phase one and the super high-risk studies, might not work so well."

Informed consent must begin with a concise and focused presentation, he continued. "That's not just the wording, it's the organization and presentation of the document." Research needs to be done on this, he said. "How do people want to see the information? What's the most important thing that participants would want to know in a phase 1a study versus a sleep study, for example?" The Secretary's Advisory Committee on Human Research Protections (SACHRP) is the only guidance researchers have, Trudeau said, adding that it is indirect because "they make recommendations to the Office for Human Research Protections, which could then be adopted as guidance."

Using Health Literacy to Inform Legal Concepts

Trudeau also raised the concept of "a reasonable person," which has been around in other legal contexts "for hundreds of years." Quoting SACHRP's commentary on the Common Rule revisions, he said:

> The reasonable person concept recognizes that it is impossible for researchers to determine what information every individual participant would

consider helpful in deciding whether or not to participate. Instead, it asks researchers to include what reasonable people in the same or similar circumstances would want to or need to know (SACHRP, 2018). Health literacy can play a role in this by helping determine what a reasonable person would understand. The reasonable person concept in law [was] developed before we had any research regarding literacy rates and health literacy research and practice, and we can learn from that to create what a reasonable person might be or know or do in various situations, through research. It's very contextual, as we have heard—it's going to be different in a cancer study versus other types of studies. So user testing and focus-group testing need to become a standard practice. That is the only way that you can really know for your specific study population what they would prefer and what would help them understand.

DISCUSSION

Assaf began the moderated discussion by emphasizing that investigators need to engage trial participants earlier in the process than they have been doing traditionally. She added that labels and package inserts can be confusing to patients, which is why "we can't wait until it's recruitment time to do something about this. We need to have potential participants involved earlier in developing materials," she said, "so we are asking questions we know they understand."

Lessons Learned from Failure

Assaf noted that during conferences and workshops, researchers and practitioners often share best practices, but less frequently share failures. "I think there's a lot we can learn from them," she said. She shared that as an investigator in the Women's Health Initiative (WHI), she and her colleagues tried many recruitment strategies for the trial, and not all of them were successful. She recounted that in this particular trial, some potential participants knew they might not personally benefit from the trial, but understood that the knowledge gained would help future generations. The recruiting relied on the altruistic nature of the trial, she added, and her team tried several print and video messages before they developed an informed consent process that potential participants could understand.

Assaf and her colleagues also found success in identifying different recruitment strategies for different populations. For recruiting African American participants, for example, they found success reaching out to pastors. For recruiting senior citizens, they found success in visiting senior centers and sharing meals with the prospective participants. The researchers also found success through a community coalition, in which volunteers recruited in their own communities for potential participants.

Assaf asked the panelists if they had any experiences in which a strategy for recruitment, informed consent, or developing lay summaries did not work, and, if so, what they learned from the experience.

Staley replied that she had previously worked for a company that aimed to match patients to clinical trials based on genomic information from their cancer tumor profile. The assumption was that messaging could be generic and "put on blast" on social media, print, radio, or the Web, and that that would take care of recruitment, she said. It seemed to her that the recruitment strategy was "filling your funnel and all of these patients will magically fall out of the bottom and be recruited and enrolled in a clinical trial," she said.

Staley and her team learned a few lessons about recruitment and enrollment quickly, she said, including the following:

- Recruitment and enrollment are about health literacy, technology literacy, and cultural literacy.
- You cannot create a single message that works for everybody.
- You have to be willing to be agile and flexible around your messaging.
- You need to be able to create a feedback loop in your recruitment and engagement process that allows for learning as you step into new communities for the first time.
- Those new communities will often share what works and what does not work for them, and if investigators do not respond in kind, they will violate the trust and respect originally offered to them.
- Before you begin building your messaging, work with communities from which you want to recruit.

She added that building relationships with communities that need help or care or new treatment options is both a requirement and a new component of cultural competence.

O'Leary agreed with Staley about the importance of messaging, adding that she had faced recruitment and retention challenges while engaged in community research at Washington University in St. Louis.

> We had some funding to create a fancy database with algorithms to enroll people from communities, to match them to open clinical trials and deliver them to the site of a trial [that] they had matched and in which they were interested. It seemed like a no-brainer. People qualified, they wanted to do it, and we took them to the door. But we *still* couldn't get them all enrolled, because the investigators couldn't figure out how to do it with folks that didn't seem to have [the resources] to get back to the site.

Successful recruitment and enrollment are really complicated, she continued, noting that her team at Washington University used that experience to improve the subsequent round of recruitment. "It's an iterative process that is never right the first time. So I think that flexibility and collaboration with the folks you're trying to reach is really the gold standard."

Trudeau explained that several years ago, he worked with a hospital association to develop a website focused on transparency. He had been "really excited" about a new gauge visual on the website that shared safety metrics at various hospitals, in which a high safety rating would read as a high percentage out of 100, resembling a speedometer. However, users interpreted the high scores negatively, because they connected it with speeding in a car. Trudeau and his team then reconfigured the visual for the website, he said, adding, "I would venture to say that every time I have user-tested a document that I've written, I have learned something."

Boulware noted that she had extensive experience in testing people's understanding of information they are given about their medical condition and also that she spent 1 year developing materials for patients with kidney disease, so she was familiar with experiencing failures and learning from them quickly. She agreed with O'Leary about health-literate messaging going beyond words, including numbers and numeracy and visual depictions. "We spend a lot of time trying to figure out how to explain a 'big difference' versus a 'small difference' to a patient," she added. "We're even thinking about how people think about French fries: small, medium, large? How do people think about magnitudes and quantities?"

User testing is a constant, she added. "I've never put a document out there that didn't need at least ten iterations to improve it, and it wasn't perfect at the end, either. I think this is evolving; we're all constantly undergoing and moving on from failures."

Assaf agreed that numeracy was an essential component of health literacy, recounting that many participants in the WHI had trouble understanding relative risk compared with absolute risk. She added that Pfizer, with help from Staley, has developed infographics and a web page that help explain the difference between absolute and relative risk for patients looking to make choices about their treatment.[4] The web page puts the concept of risk into context, she said, for example, crossing the street versus getting into an airplane.

---

[4] To view some of Pfizer's infographics, see www.pfizer.com/MedicineSafety (accessed September 18, 2019) and to view Pfizer's web page on understanding risk, see www.pfizer.com/products/patient-safety/Making-Good-Treatment-Choices/Understanding-Risk (accessed September 18, 2019).

Strategies for Sharing Trial Results

Olayinka Shiyanbola from the University of Wisconsin–Madison School of Pharmacy expressed her appreciation for each of the panelists' presentations. She asked two questions:

1. What are some other strategies for distributing results at the end of a trial?
2. What are some strategies for sharing information with people who have reading difficulties or are unable to read the trial summary?

O'Leary replied that there is a focus on lay summaries because they are a regulatory requirement. Because of the nature of some large or cross-continental trials, she said, the summaries are already not necessarily the best approach to sharing information, just the required one. She continued

> I also don't think [lay summaries] are bad. It's important that participants have a piece of paper that is readable that they can find online or get from their doctor's office. It's good support for conversation and understanding, and it's an easy box to check off, that everybody received one—it's a good start. But in community-based research, investigators often try to gather initial groups of participants, discuss what happened, and use it as an opportunity to think about what's next and what was missing. Based on feedback from research participants, some investigators have started writing scientific papers that are published in journals and go on your CV, as well as another version that is more public facing, and is published in a newspaper or in a neighborhood newsletter. I hear that participants really like those. I think some of the advocates here might agree that they would want to be engaged all the way through the process and that includes deciding at the end [and after] how we describe the trial itself.
>
> Video is always great; it's just so expensive. I have found that researchers don't have a lot of money on the back end of a trial to pay for a complicated production, so you have to figure out what your investment is going to be: is it worth more for you to have a video that everyone can see, or to have deep engagement with a smaller group? Those are all choices that reflect the philosophy and values connected with the community and the trial.

Boulware added that at Duke, she is developing an information portal where study participants can log in at the beginning of the trial, and have constant communication with the investigative teams throughout the entire journey. This option is limited because it requires access to technology, she noted, but it will enhance communication for many participants, including at the end of the study.

Assaf said that she had held small group sessions at the ends of the trials she had worked on, especially for particularly vulnerable populations. The participants would come and have snacks and meet with others who had participated in the trial, she said, and the research team would run a presentation, explain the results, take questions, and generally make themselves available to chat with participants about any questions or concerns they had. "Obviously everyone can't do that," she added, "but it was really powerful and impactful to do it."

Ensuring Comprehension in Participants with Lower Health Literacy

Michael Wolf from the Feinberg School of Medicine at Northwestern University asked the panelists what they recommended to ensure patient comprehension among patients with lower health literacy. He said that in his experience, incorporating tools like "teach-back" helped improve participants' comprehension and retention of information, but he added that incorporating some health literacy tools seemed like a deterrent for some participants, because it took up more of their time. He added that "no matter how good the written material is, it will not do anything for people with the lowest levels of health literacy. They are not going to utilize it."

Trudeau agreed, adding that he believed informed consent should be a memorialization of the education that has occurred between participants and investigators, not just a transactional document to be signed. "I do think that the Common Rule revision is supporting this shift toward facilitating understanding, using teach back, and a whole planned educational process, not just the 'consent process,'" he said.

Boulware echoed Trudeau, adding that she has often thought that investigators seem to race to get informed consent signatures, but wondered if the consent process should actually be broken up into separate pieces. She continued:

> Do we need to ensure a person understands Part A before they can get to Part B and Part C? The chances of decisional regret at the end are much lower when a participant has had time to really digest what it means to participate in the study.

Retaining Participants with Lower Health Literacy

Wolf described a meta-analysis about AIDS studies, which concluded that patients with lower health literacy are "significantly more likely to not be retained, which puts a huge skew on a lot of the scientific evidence we even know about these groups."[5] He continued, "What do we do to make sure that patients with low health literacy aren't marginalized?"

O'Leary replied that in her previous work in community research, she worked on HIV prevention among women who used drugs. "We lost participants left and right, for a lot of reasons," she said, but the way she and her colleagues were able to find people again was by reaching out in person, referring again to Boulware's comments about home visits.

> I would call and say, "This is Catina, I haven't seen you in 16 months, and your information is really important to me. I want to know how you're doing and how this worked for you. Do you mind if I drop by?" Nobody ever said no. They were always so happy when I showed up at their house; it was a really big deal that somebody cared enough to come to their house. And then they would call back for the next one. They would never miss a follow-up again after that. I kept the same number for about 14 years even after I wasn't in the same office at Washington University, because people would call and say "I was in a study a long time ago and it was really great. I just wonder what you are all doing now."
>
> That effort to connect is so meaningful and transformational that I think we should figure out how to do it more. The hard part is figuring out how to build in enough funding to cover that all the way through. I think a lot of studies just don't have the financial support to keep that going, and of course, not every interviewer can make home visits.

Staley added that, from a patient perspective, clinical trials are very specific in the sense that everyone prepares for one trial at a time. Investigators may be recruiting from the same populations but behave differently when reaching out to communities, she continued. "If there was a way for more industry collaboration around therapeutic areas or disease states where you're working for the collective good educating the community, not only about clinical trials, but health in general, we do a better service for everyone in general."

"Reasonable Person"

Consuelo H. Wilkins from the Meharry–Vanderbilt Alliance cautioned the panelists and workshop audience to be careful using the term "reasonable person." She added:

---

[5] The abstract "Exploring the Impact of Low Health Literacy on Participant Attrition in Clinical Research Studies" was authored by L. M. Curtis, A. Federman, R. O'Conor, M. Martynenko, E. Friesmema, S. Persell, and M. S. Wolf and presented by L. M. Curtis at the Health Literacy Annual Research Conference in Bethesda, Maryland, in October 2015.

For me, "reasonable person" is a phrase used from the standpoint of the people who have power and privilege. That can mean that we are missing the people who we want in our trials who don't have power and privilege.

Trudeau agreed that Wilkins was "absolutely right," adding it has been a concern for a long time. In the nonresearch world of consent, the "reasonable person" standard applies in about half the states in the United States, he said, but the problem is that

> the standard has been developed for privileged folks, privileged judges, privileged juries. I think the health literacy community now has some research showing who "reasonable people" are, which is not necessarily privileged folks with an education and degree from a prestigious university. I hope we can expand the meaning of the term because, as a legal standard, it should apply to the majority of folks.

Health Literacy Metrics

Wilkins, along with Becky Williams from the National Library of Medicine, both asked the panelists about the right health literacy metrics for participants and trials, how to capture them, and how the goal of health-literate practices might compete with the goal of enrolling participants in a study.

Staley replied that she has explored this idea, noting that smoking cessation and weight loss programs often use 22 questions in a clinical setting to evaluate the readiness of a patient for the program. She added she has wondered why trials do not use the same types of questions before participants are in the informed consent stage,

> to ensure that they are at a point where they understand what's needed in general to participate in clinical research. I don't think we do enough to assess the patient from that kind of perspective because there are financial implications to participating in clinical research. There's time away from work. There is a whole host of things that the patient has to consider that are not addressed during informed consent. I've never seen an informed consent document that says "you need to be away from work 5 days a week for 1 hour" or "you will need to take time off from work and drive to the hospital 2 hours away." We never really consider those kinds of questions and I think we have to focus on the participant's context before we even get to informed consent. And the education has to be continuous.

Staley added that patient fatigue is an important consideration too. O'Leary replied that one of the golden rules of health literacy is to engage people early and often in everything you do, and if you do that, the outcomes are different. She noted that authenticity was a part of meaningful engagement among investigators and participants, but added that it would be impossible to develop documents that were specific enough to address a participant needing to leave their job for a few hours. That, she continued, would be where the investigators come in to support the regulatory document and ensure that participants understand what they are signing up for. Regarding metrics, she said, she was not sure about the best ones for everything, but noted that even though "adherence" and "compliance" were not health-literate terms, they are often proxies for how much people understand and engage, and thus were still relevant.

Patient Portals

Collyar asked the panelists for their thoughts or experiences around the use of patient portals in trials or clinical settings.

The burden is on the patient to ensure continuity of care by carrying their medical information between clinical research and primary care providers (PCPs), said Staley, and "it's a nightmare." Referring to her own experience as a cancer patient, she said:

> I've told my oncologist and PCP that they can't retire until I do, because they know my story. I've made a conscious decision to stay with the same health care team because I actually feel that having the longevity that I've had with my oncology and primary care team has made me healthier and safer as a patient than going from one system to another. Yes, I seek out second or third opinions, and I always return to my primary care physician and my oncologist, because as long as they are the center of truth for my health care story, I feel confident in that.
>
> But I'm the one carrying records and connecting information sets about my journey when I need to make a decision, and I think my challenge to industry is to develop a central source for the patient who wants to participate in trials that might be with different sponsors or pharmaceutical companies. If I'm on a pharma company A trial, and then enroll in a pharma company B trial, I want continuity of my clinical research journey available to the researchers, not just data points of a very specific moment in time.
>
> How can industry build this framework to allow for seamless information exchange and allow for continuous educational processes throughout so the patients, physicians, and researchers are constantly learning and evolving?

The Importance of Building Trust and Relationships

Patty Spears from the University of North Carolina Lineberger Patient Research Advocacy Group said that she believes the paradigm of clinical trials needs to be flipped to be patient-focused, instead of trial-focused. "It's a partnership where you build a relationship, and then you focus on what trial is best for the patient, not which trial you are pushing today," she said. There are a lot of different people involved in this process, she continued, including patients, clinicians, and research professionals, but "the number one reason why patients enroll in clinical trials is because their physician asked them to."

Terry C. Davis from the Louisiana State University Health Sciences Center reiterated that relationships between patients and providers were important, and that includes clinical research assistants. She asked O'Leary about user reactions to the table O'Leary showed.

O'Leary replied that there were many iterations of the HLM informed consent form, starting with the original draft from Janssen. She said that HLM tested it with more than 100 people during the first round, and continued to make changes through several focus groups. "I don't think there's a standard application," she added, and the graphics, tables, colors, charts, and lines will require participation to test every one, every time.

Boulware added that, as a general internist, she felt that PCPs were often left out of the clinical trials process with regard to their patients. She said that despite playing a key role in trial participants' care, PCPs frequently have little information about the actual trials.

Boulware said that PCPs should be thoughtfully integrated into the process of clinical trials, developing an understanding of the role of the PCP, and how they can continue to help their patients throughout the trial. It was exciting to hear PCPs included in the conversation, she said, but it will be difficult in practice if they are never actually prepared to help patients with trials.

Davis added that many PCPs she had worked with were from federally qualified health centers and did not have time to search for clinical trials that would be appropriate for their patients. Many rural PCPs are unfamiliar with academic researchers, which is also a hindrance, she said. "If we want PCPs to help us [as investigators]," she said, "we've got to make it easy for them to find out about appropriate trials to mention to their patients. We need relationships—trust is everything."

Assaf agreed, adding that PCPs could really benefit from having health-literate information (with brief talking points, for example) to share with patients. She also noted that a particularly delicate time for trial participants is when the results of a trial are made public; some of the results may startle participants. If PCPs are notified about these results ahead of time, they can counsel the participants on the best decision to make for their care around stopping or changing a drug.

Lawrence G. Smith from the Donald and Barbara Zucker School of Medicine at Hofstra/Northwell and Northwell Health added that trust between PCPs and patients is at the root of successful patient understanding and treatment, and developing that trust is an ongoing process.

O'Leary said that printed materials are a necessary supplement to a structured conversation with patients and trial participants.

Regarding the trial process and, specifically, informed consent, Staley said:

> Everything is a race. We're in a race for the patient's signature on informed consent. We're in a race to bring a new drug to market. We're in a race all about speed. It's got to be faster, and it's got to be cheaper. It's got to be done yesterday.
>
> But what we're talking about is the fact that we have to stop, take time to build relationships, and take time to process information. The system is built around speed, and making decisions in this rapid-fire mindset. It's very hard to slow it down; it feels almost counterintuitive.

She added that there is a dichotomy between the clinical care side and the clinical research side of medicine.

> If you're focused on clinical care, your focus is to deliver care to the patient at that very moment. If you're focused on clinical research, you're looking at the end goal: does this therapy work or not? A patient sits in the middle and doesn't look at it as clinical care or clinical research. They look at it as health care. They look at it as getting better or staying well.
>
> We can go a long way in helping patients understand that there are subtle differences between the two worlds, but let's find a way to begin building bridges that allow for the health care journey to be as seamless as possible for the patient. We've got the tools. We have the technology. It's about building the relationships at this point.

Referring to Smith's point about the process of developing trust, Trudeau said, "it made me think about the European Medicines Agency having a regulation that requires conversations for informed consent." The conversation is not just in writing; it is a requirement that helps you build trust with participants, he added.

In terms of informed consent, he said,

> we shouldn't be thinking about this as one document, maybe "talk about the study and sign," and then "talk about the risk and sign," and continue

with different conversations. It might not be something you can do logistically for low-risk studies but for the really high-risk first-in-human studies, this seems like something that needs to be embedded into the culture of what we do during the educational process. And if the lawyers need signatures, that's fine, but we'll get them on different days.

Phyllis J. Pettit Nassi from the University of Utah Huntsman Cancer Institute explained that part of her responsibility in her program is to do outreach to rural frontier populations, including American Indian and Alaska Native farmers, ranchers, polygamists, and Hutterites. She added that clinical trials are a component of the health education programs she runs, and they are included along a continuum of patient experiences. Pettit Nassi believes that we need to restructure how we speak about clinical trials so that people understand that trials are a part of the health care system and the patient experience. She noted that people cannot access something that they have never heard of and do not know about. She also suggested relating clinical trials to people or experiences that are familiar. She added that she often mentions former President Jimmy Carter's participation in a clinical trial as an example of someone who is in a trial but still active and engaged with other activities.

Staley said that she would like to see the health care system move from reactive to proactive. "Every health care interaction I've had since I was 19 years old was reactive in nature," she said, "from the first moment I was diagnosed with cancer. It's been that way ever since. We can't continue to work in this reactive mode."

Jennifer Dillaha from the Arkansas Department of Health commented that she saw clinical trials as an opportunity to support patients toward increasing their health literacy. "It seems that a clinical trial would be a wonderful opportunity to coach patients, empower them, and develop trust, so by the time the patient finished the clinical trial, their health literacy skills would be much more robust than when they started," she said.

Behtash Bahador from the Center for Information and Study on Clinical Research Participation asked how professionals from academia, industry, clinical practice, and research have navigated engaging trial participants in a health-literate manner while still dealing with the operational need for expediency.

Boulware, speaking as a National Institutes of Health (NIH)-funded investigator, replied that she found there to be several issues around funding for such practices. Typically, she said, investigators are expected to begin enrolling participants as soon as the funding is granted, making it difficult for investigators to do any pretrial work of engaging communities and potential participants. She added that NIH Clinical Translational Science Awards (CTSA) support community engagement by providing some financial support, but they are rather underfunded. At the Duke University Clinical & Translational Science Institute, which Boulware directs, the community engagement core is their largest, but it shares its funding with 14 other cores.[6] To accommodate this type of pretrial community engagement that occurs before, during, and after a study's standard funding timeline, Boulware continued, the entire mechanism of funding needs to change.

As a final comment from the panelists, O'Leary explained that her earlier career focused on community-engaged research. She noted that those studies had community-engagement strategies built in, so funding was structured accordingly. The broader trial industry has not picked it up, she said, but "it's not impractical." Wrapping up the discussion, she continued:

> Advocates want to be included before a trial is even funded and to think about research questions. They want to be engaged—not just regarding the research question, but the logistics questions, as well. I think those models from community-engaged research can be more broadly utilized. It can be uncomfortable and complicated, and it is a real challenge to the scientific model as many people know and understand it. But I think it works. Investigators will have to be really thoughtful about what their intentions are and who their audience is and what their purpose is.

REFERENCES

Boulware, L. E., P. L. Ephraim, J. Ameling, L. Lewis-Boyer, H. Rabb, R. C. Greer, D. C. Crews, B. G. Jaar, P. Auguste, T. S. Purnell, J. A. Lamprea-Monteleagre, T. Olufade, L. Gimenez, C. Cook, T. Campbell, A. Woodall, H. Ramamurthi, C. A. Davenport, K. R. Choudhury, M. R. Weir, D. S. Hanes, N. Y. Wang, H. Vilme, and N. R. Powe. 2018. Effectiveness of informational decision aids and a live donor financial assistance program on pursuit of live kidney transplants in African American hemodialysis patients. *BMC Nephrology* 19(1):107. https://doi.org/10.1186/s12882-018-0901-x.

Boulware, L. E., P. L. Ephraim, F. Hill-Briggs, D. L. Roter, L. R. Bone, J. L. Wolff, L. Lewis-Boyer, D. M. Levine, R. C. Greer, D. C. Crews, K. A. Gudzune, M. C. Albert, H. C. Ramamurthi, J. M. Ameling, C. A. Davenport, H.-J. Lee, J. F. Pendergast, N.-Y. Wang, K. A. Carson, V. Sneed, D. J. Gayles, S. J. Flynn, D. Monroe, D. Hickman, L. Purnell, M. Simmons, A. Fisher, N. DePasquale, J. Charleston, H. J. Aboutamar, A. N. Cabacungan, and L. A. Cooper. 2020. Hypertension self-management in socially disadvantaged African Americans: The Achieving Blood Pressure Control Together (ACT) randomized comparative effectiveness trial. *Journal of General Internal Medicine* 35(1):142–152. doi: 10.1007/s11606-019-05396-7.

GPO (U.S. Government Printing Office). 2017. Federal policy for the protection of human subjects. *Federal Register* 82:7149. https://www.govinfo.gov/content/pkg/FR-2017-01-19/pdf/2017-01058.pdf (accessed January 25, 2020).

---

[6] For more information about CTSA cores at Duke University's Clinical & Translational Science Institute, see https://www.ctsi.duke.edu/about/ctsa-cores (accessed September 19, 2019).

SACHRP (Secretary's Advisory Committee on Human Research Protections). 2018. *Attachment C—New "key information" informed consent requirements*. SACHRP, October 17, 2018. https://www.hhs.gov/ohrp/sachrp-committee/recommendations/attachment-c-november-13-2018/index.html (accessed September 17, 2019).

Strigo, T. S., P. L. Ephraim, I. Pounds, F. Hill-Briggs, L. Darrell, M. Ellis, D. Sudan, H. Rabb, D. Segev, N.-Y. Wang, M. Kaiser, M. Falkovic, J. F. Lebov, and L. E. Boulware. 2015. The TALKS study to improve communication, logistical, and financial barriers to live donor kidney transplantation in African Americans: Protocol of a randomized clinical trial. *BMC Nephrology* 16(160). https://doi.org/10.1186/s12882-015-0153-y.

Trunomi and CommVault. 2018. *GPDR FAQs*. https://eugdpr.org/the-regulation/gdpr-faqs (accessed September 17, 2019).

4

Experiences Implementing Health Literacy Best Practices in Clinical Trials

The next panel of the workshop featured three speakers who presented their programs or research on implementing health literacy practices in clinical trials. Connie Arnold, professor of medicine, Louisiana State University (LSU) Health Sciences Center, described her takeaways from implementing two different health literacy interventions to promote cancer screenings. Lauren McCormack, vice president of the Public Health Research Division at RTI International, then spoke about her research on making clinical trials and informed consent more patient centered. Finally, Saira Z. Sheikh, assistant professor of medicine at the University of North Carolina (UNC) at Chapel Hill, director of the UNC Rheumatology Lupus Clinic, and director of the Clinical Trials Program at UNC's Thurston Arthritis Research Center, addressed some common barriers to patient participation in clinical trials. Phyllis J. Pettit Nassi, associate director of Research and Science, Special Populations at the Huntsman Cancer Institute, moderated a discussion between the speakers and the audience.

LESSONS LEARNED FROM TWO HEALTH LITERACY INTERVENTIONS TO IMPROVE COLORECTAL CANCER SCREENINGS

Connie Arnold, Professor of Medicine,
Louisiana State University Health Sciences Center

Arnold opened her presentation describing two clinical trials that she and Terry C. Davis had directed, during which they implemented health literacy interventions in cancer screenings in mostly rural areas.

The First Trial: 2007 to 2012

The first study was conducted between 2007 and 2012, observing eight federally qualified health centers' (FQHCs') colorectal cancer (CRC) screenings. Arnold noted that before she and Davis write grant proposals, they call the chief executive officers (CEOs) of the FQHCs they want to work with, set up a meeting, and go to meet them. Together, they walk through what works in the clinic for patients, and ask the staff how they envision any interventions progressing. "As Terry [Davis] always tells me, it's all about the relationship," she continued, "especially when you're implementing interventions in a clinic you don't actually work at." Additionally, she said, clinic staff can advise investigators about what interventions might work really well or really poorly with patients.

Arnold also noted that FQHCs and community clinics and their staff are often unaccustomed to the cycle of grant proposals in clinical research. She continued:

> If you don't get funded the first time, you resubmit your proposal a year and a half, or maybe two years later. One of the keys is to keep the clinics involved in the process. We are very clear and very upfront with them about what we are submitting, and what we plan to resubmit, how long the proposals take to be reviewed, and we keep them updated on the status and the results of reviews. That's really important, because otherwise, they forget who you are.

The FQHCs, she added, are government-supported clinics that provide health care services for up to 28 million people, regardless of their insurance status (HRSA, 2019). They are generally located in areas that are medically underserved, she said, so the target for the trial was five FQHCs in northern Louisiana, which is a predominantly rural area.

Arnold went on to explain that the first study was made of up 67 percent African American patients and 32 percent white patients, with 56 percent of them reading below an eighth-grade level (Arnold et al., 2016a,b; Davis et al., 2013, 2014a,b, 2015a,b). Additionally, the investigators had built focus groups into the study design to include patients and providers in developing and testing materials like brochures and surveys. One of the changes the investigators made to the materials involved developing a Likert scale but shaped vertically, because it improved comprehension for patients with lower health literacy. They also used something they called the "two-step" process, to encourage patients to identify the degree to which they agreed or disagreed with a statement on the scale. Arnold had found that patients with lower health literacy rarely answered that they "strongly" agreed or disagreed with any of the survey statements, so she had the research assistants (RAs) start the question with "do you agree or disagree?" and then ask a follow-up question to define the answer. For example, if the patient said they agreed with the statement, the RA would ask them to clarify if they agreed or strongly agreed, which helped encourage more accurate responses.

The investigators also developed short videos with patients, she continued, using their interests and experiences to show a woman receiving a mammogram for a breast cancer screening and a man getting a fecal occult blood test (FOBT) for a CRC screening. She added that they used stock photos in the first brochures they developed, but in the subsequent study, they used actual patient photos. "We tried to incorporate all of the principles we know about health literacy," she said, to find out what would resonate with the population. She added that, as great as they felt the videos were, patients did not really want to watch them. The three-arm study involved the following:

1. An enhanced usual-care arm: patient given information, recommendation, no-cost mammogram or FOBT kit, and suggestion to talk with a primary care physician (PCP)
2. A health-literate care arm: patient given information, recommendation, no-cost mammogram or FOBT with simple instructions, pamphlet, video, and suggestion to talk with a PCP
3. A health-literate care-plus-nurse (plus) arm: patient given information, recommendation, nurse case manager, tailored education, either a mammogram scheduled by a nurse or an FOBT kit, and a follow-up call to remind and problem solve

The investigators also hired an RA for the clinics. To enroll three or four or five patients per week, Arnold said, they did not require a full-time RA, but the investigators worked with the FQHC CEOs to train someone to do informed consent, distribute materials, or run the questionnaire. Most of the time, the clinics chose a staff member who already had some extra time, Arnold said.

In 2007, Arnold added, the intervention really affected CRC screening knowledge, more than mammography and breast cancer knowledge (Arnold et al., 2009, 2017). The investigators were unsurprised that the results revealed that the patients in the health-literate care and the plus arms had a significant improvement in colon cancer screenings—the clinics had between 1 and 3 percent screening rates when the investigators began the study, she said. She noted that in years two and three, patients did not always return to the clinic to get their FOBT screening kit. The clinic mailed the kits to patients in every arm, but it was a challenge to have patients understand that they needed to return the kit every year, she explained.

Arnold noted that there were a handful of challenges she had identified when working with the FQHC partners:

- Community clinics focus on service for patients, not research fidelity.
- It can be difficult to find qualified RAs in rural areas.
- Hiring RAs from clinic staff is a "catch-22"—while their relationships are helpful to the work overall, research is usually their secondary job and is put on the back burner if the clinic is understaffed.
- There is high physician turnover in rural areas.
- Follow-up calls are feasible, but phone lines are commonly disconnected then reconnected. The calls are often time consuming and it was not cost-effective to hire a nurse.
- Patients lose FOBT kits or forget to complete them.
- The wait time for diagnostic colonoscopy at LSU was up to 1 year during this study.

The Second Trial: 2012 Through 2018

For the second study, Arnold said, the investigators used what they learned in the first one: health literacy information was going to be standard in both arms, because they knew that it was more effective. "There wasn't any reason to go back to using enhanced usual care," she said. With colon cancer screenings, the issue was largely years two and three, in that patients did not continue to use the FOBT kits. "The point of our second study," she continued, "was to look at automated and personal phone calls. Did it make a difference if it was a live person or would an automated phone call be just as effective?" The investigators worked again with clinic staff, this time in southern Louisiana. They also created a recorded phone call with a person who had a southern Louisiana accent, she noted.

The second study, which began in 2012, used the fecal immunochemical test (FIT) instead of the FOBT for CRC screenings, though both still required yearly tests, Arnold noted.[1] At the time, she said, rural clinics were not referring patients for colonoscopies, because they were unlikely to be able to pay for them. The investigators simplified the FIT instructions and colorectal cancer screening materials and everyone enrolled in the trial was given health-literate materials by an RA in the clinic, Arnold explained. They had hired RAs in the same manner as in the first study, she added, and the RAs demonstrated the FIT, which could be confusing.

---

[1] For information about FIT, FOBT, and colonoscopy screenings, see www.cancer.org/cancer/colon-rectal-cancer/detection-diagnosis-staging/screening-tests-used.html (accessed September 20, 2019).

However, years two and three bore the same issues as the first study. If a patient did not return their FIT kit within 4 weeks of the first appointment, they received a follow-up call. Patients were randomized to receive either a personal call or an automated call. During years two and three, the FIT kits were mailed to patients, with a reminder letter preceding it. Arnold noted that the investigators were sure to brand the letters and packages with the name of the clinic as well as LSU to remind patients receiving them that they were part of the study, and to emphasize that the PCPs at the clinic felt it was important.

In years two and three, patients required more phone call reminders (Arnold et al., 2019; Davis et al., 2019). However, she noted, the automated call worked just as well as the personal call. Older patients preferred the personal call, she said, but overall, the calls were equally effective. Arnold shared a list of the lessons and challenges from the second study:

- Regulatory paperwork was a barrier for community clinic RAs.
- RAs need concrete research instructions and frequent "teach-back" of protocol.
- Frequent face-to-face clinic visits build relationships and enhance fidelity.
- Arranging for diagnostic colonoscopies for the uninsured was challenging.

She also described what approaches and considerations she thought were needed going forward and why:

- **Creative approaches are needed to promote long-term screening.**
  o Offer screening options and use decision aids to help patients identify the CRC test that they find most acceptable and feasible.
  o Use text or automated calls to remind patients to compete the test.
- **The environment has changed.**
  o When we began this grant, none of the clinics had electronic health records, and now they all have them.
  o Louisiana has now taken Medicaid expansion, so having a colonoscopy is a reality for patients in rural areas.
  o Because of Medicaid expansion, more gastroenterologists are having clinics in rural areas for 1 or 2 days per week. More rural hospitals are offering colonoscopies.

MAKING CLINICAL TRIALS AND INFORMED CONSENT MORE PATIENT-CENTERED

Lauren McCormack, Vice President,
Public Health Research Division, RTI International

McCormack expressed her thanks to her colleagues at RTI, as well as to external collaborators, for their involvement in the work she was presenting at the workshop. She explained that she would be sharing some of the patient-centered strategies that RTI is implementing with UNC, Duke University, and Vanderbilt University. She continued, identifying several elements of what is currently not working with informed consent in trials (see Box 4-1) as well as several initiatives to improve patient experiences and the informed consent process.

Initiatives to Improve Patient Experiences

Several studies have examined the process of improving the consent experience, she added, as well as outcomes and measurements related to comprehension. For example, Beskow and colleagues (2017) and Grady and colleagues (2017) both found that a simplified version of a consent form was "just as good" as the standard consent form in practice, she said, though Beskow and colleagues did find that the simplified version was not superior for participants with lower health literacy. "One of the things I think we really need to be focusing on is looking at subgroup analyses and not just looking at everyone as a whole," she continued. In another study, Kim and Kim (2015) found that a simplified consent form was associated with higher levels of objective and subjective understanding, she said, the

---

BOX 4-1
Current Challenges Related to Informed Consent

- Lack of bidirectional communication
- Overwhelming participants with forms
- Participants signing consent forms without completely understanding the information
- Participant misunderstanding of the rationale and design of the study, particularly randomization, leading to higher dropout rates

SOURCE: Adapted from a presentation by Lauren McCormack at the workshop Health Literacy in Clinical Trials: Practice and Impact on April 11, 2019.

"objective being scoring questions as correct or incorrect, which is how we measured understanding in the study being presented."

The use of interactive technology, she said, also has the potential to improve the process, but "it comes with its own set of complications and challenges and it often cannot replace the human connection. The question is, how do we still obtain that human interaction and connection but without the cost and time generally involved in one-on-one patient interactions?"

McCormack recommended paying attention to the Clinical Trials Transformation Initiative (CTTI), explaining that it is a public–private partnership of about 75 different organizations. CTTI, she said, has made recommendations recently about improving the informed consent process, as well as areas of patient engagement (CTTI, 2019a,b). She added that CTTI has general recommendations along with specific recommendations, such as how to tier the consent form (CTTI, 2019a).

> Their tiering process suggests putting the federally required content up front, which would be HIPAA [Health Insurance Portability and Accountability Act] language followed by the IRB [Institutional Review Board]-required content. Their example is in chapters, well organized using health literacy principles with an introduction or summary of the trial.

McCormack added that CTTI has also recommended training those who facilitate informed consent processes as well as the use of a discussion tool to help participants with understanding (CTTI, 2019a). She also noted that the U.S. Food and Drug Administration (FDA) has used its patient-focused drug development initiative to identify approaches to facilitating patient involvement and minimizing patient burden.[2] The primary focus of the initiative is to better incorporate the patient's voice in drug development and evaluation. One element of this initiative is conducting "trade-off studies using discrete choice analyses or patient preference studies" to understand patient preference with respect to balancing benefits and risks. FDA has also published electronic informed consent (eIC) guidance, she noted (FDA, 2016).

Several different pharmaceutical industry and tech industry groups are now focused on the last issue of eIC, she noted, adding, "I would like to encourage all of us to coordinate and share lessons learned."

---

[2] For more information about the FDA patient-focused drug development initiative, see https://www.fda.gov/drugs/development-approval-process-drugs/cder-patient-focused-drug-development (accessed January 13, 2020).

A Randomized Controlled Trial to Assess the Efficacy of an Informed Consent Tool

The Importance of Decision Aids

"This brings me to the value of decision aids," McCormack said, explaining that the Cochrane Collaboration has published several systematic reviews that emphasize "the importance of personalized decision making; providing tailored information to people that allows them to consider their preferences and values; and looking at outcomes such as knowledge and decisional conflict" (Stacey et al., 2017). McCormack noted that RTI carefully considers this research when developing decision aids.

Informed Consent Tool Trial

McCormack's team conducted a randomized controlled trial to assess the efficacy of an informed consent tool, and specifically to address two questions:

1. Does the tool improve the capacity of individuals to make an informed decision about consenting relative to standard practice?
2. Is there variation in the tool's utility by level of cognitive function?

The hypothesis, McCormack said, was that there may be a threshold at which a tool is more beneficial, and below which a tool may not make a significant difference. The trial participants were individuals with fragile X syndrome, ages 12 through 40. The study design based its measures on the MacArthur Competence Assessment Tool for Clinical Research (Appelbaum, 2008), she said, focusing on whether the participants

1. **understand** the nature of the trial and its procedures,
2. **appreciate** the impact of participating in the trial on their own care,
3. use **reasoning** to decide whether they will participate, and
4. **express a choice** about participating in the trial.

The trial itself was hypothetical, so participants never enrolled after the decision, McCormack added. She noted that they developed their informed consent tool using strategies like plain language and clear communication. "Interactive engagement was emphasized and we used multimedia communication," she said. They also conducted a values clarification exercise, in which an avatar narrates to the trial participant and walks them through the informed consent process, all in a first-grade reading level. They developed several different avatars, she said, that can be selected based on the needs of the study and its participants—they can vary by age, culture, ethnicity, gender, literacy level, and spoken language (American Sign Language is also available).

The informed consent modules included Institutional Review Board–required elements, McCormack explained, including the study purpose, what the study involves and how it works, risks and benefits, and the participants' ability to withdraw from the study. She noted that these were standard, but some trials might have additional needs and modules. There were a few benefits to using the module, she added. Investigators could transform content to lower reading-grade levels and explain complex design elements or technology, but the tool also standardized the presentation of the information. Because there were participants in multiple study sites, having the information standardized helped protect the participants and the researchers, she said.

McCormack then explained that the participants received a score on a scale of zero to 100, to compare the informed consent tool with the comparison group. Taken as a whole, the full sample ($n = 89$) did not show any greater understanding after exposure to the consent tool. Once the sample was categorized by cognitive impairment, however, it became clear that there was improvement in understanding among the less cognitively impaired (higher IQ) participants. These individuals showed significant improvement in understanding, McCormack said. She noted that there was no improvement among those with higher cognitive impairment (lower IQ), but that was expected by the researchers.

McCormack added that her team has published several manuscripts about this study, including the protocol, the process of developing a decision-support tool, and its impact on decisional capacity. Several populations may benefit from decision aids, she said, particularly populations with cognitive impairments or intellectual disabilities; pediatric and adolescent populations; populations with sporadic or limited ties to the health care system; and populations with lower education or health literacy.

McCormack explained that RTI is working on infusing health literacy at the enrollment stage by

- training research coordinators,
- developing and distributing frequently asked questions and other take-home materials, and
- bringing in a study advisory committee (which is partially made up of patients) to review and provide feedback on all patient-facing materials.

Citing a recent *Health Affairs* article, McCormack closed her talk by noting that the percentage of people who said their health care providers involve them in health care decisions as much as they would like has increased from 51.6 percent in 2007 to 56.8 percent—a slight but important uptick (Brach, 2019).

CRITICAL CONVERSATIONS IN CLINICAL TRIALS

Saira Z. Sheikh, Director, Clinical Trials Program, University of North Carolina Thurston Arthritis Research Center

Sheikh opened her talk by reiterating that there is a need to infuse health literacy practices into every step of the clinical trials process, and she wanted to start with the critical conversations that need to occur "well before" a patient decides to participate in a trial.

When, Where, and How?

Sheikh focuses on the "when, where, and how" of conversations about clinical trials between patients and providers, she said. As a rheumatologist and allergist immunologist, Sheikh has "a lot" of conversations with patients about clinical trials—not just because she cares about advancing science, she added, but because there is a critical need for newer and better therapies for her patients. Evidently, she said, this is a good thing, because "the majority of patients who participate in a clinical trial learn about it from their provider" (NIH, 2016). Regarding the backdrop against which such conversations occur, she added that health literacy demands are placed on patients "as soon as they set foot in the hospital or clinic." Signs, directions, and paperwork can be overwhelming, and the clinics are often busy, with limited time slots for patients. These factors can be stressful and confusing for anyone, let alone for someone with lower health literacy, she added.

From the patients' perspectives, this often feels like an overload of information:

> It's difficult to understand and process: often, patients are learning about a new diagnosis, there is disease prognosis, there is medication, there is dosage information, and there are costs. And then there are all these other factors—family, culture, beliefs, and it's even more difficult for patients with limited English proficiency.

The questions she receives from colleagues and physicians across the country, she said, are "so in the middle of all of this, when, where, and how are we supposed to have conversations about clinical trials? Is this a good time? If not, when is a good time?" It does not surprise her, she said, and addition to African Americans. She noted that she is leading a longitudinal study in an underserved area in Durham, North Carolina, while a colleague is co-leading a sister study in an underserved area in Rochester, New York, to test the real-world effectiveness of the model.

Patient Advocates for Lupus Studies

The Patient Advocates for Lupus Studies (PALS) program is funded by Lupus Therapeutics and the Lupus Research Alliance through the lupus clinical investigators network. Other project partners are KDH Research and Communication, and Sheikh's co-principal investigator for the project is at Emory University. The PALS program is an early educational intervention to introduce clinical trials to individuals before they have to decide if they want to participate. It is a peer-to-peer communication program, which has been particularly effective in engaging communities with the health care system, Sheikh said, but it has not been applied specifically to populations of patients with lupus in clinical trials.

In a survey of 300 lupus patients, when asked what would motivate them to participate in a clinical trial, more than 80 percent of respondents said that talking with other patients who have taken part in a clinical trial would have made them very likely to participate, Sheikh reported. Because of this, the PALS program was designed as a peer-support and educational intervention, and individuals living with lupus would be trained to serve as "trial agnostic resources" for patients. Principal investigators, evaluators, and patient advocate facilitators participated in a live training session, the materials of which were developed with input from patients living with lupus.

The PALS program has trained patient advocates who conduct semi-structured educational sessions, including introductions, clinical trials basics, decision making and risks and benefits, informed consent and patient protections, and patient-specific barriers and concerns. As part of the study, Sheikh said, they are looking to measure clinical trial knowledge, satisfaction with the program, intentions, and attitudes toward clinical trials. In terms of behavior, she said, the best predictor is the patient's intention to perform that particular behavior.

Programs to Address Unmet Needs and Promote Representation of All Participants in Lupus Clinical Trials Using Mobile Technology for Engagement

Sheikh explained that the last program she wanted to talk about is referred to as Project PURPLE (Programs to Address Unmet Needs and

Promote Representation of All Participants in Lupus Clinical Trials Using Mobile Technology for Engagement), and its project partners include RTI International and Pattern Health. The program has four main areas of focus:

1. Culturally tailored materials for all literacy levels and personalization
2. Animations that explain complex study concepts
3. Interactive decision-support activities
4. Knowledge assessment surveys, based on teach-back principles

Sheikh explained that because 6 billion of the world's 7 billion people have mobile phones they do not need to make a case for using mobile technology for any specific intervention (UN, 2013). In fact, she said, smartphones are helping to bridge gaps among African Americans, Hispanics, and white Americans. African Americans and Hispanics are more likely to rely on a smartphone to review or research health information (Perrin and Turner, 2019; Vangeepuram et al., 2018). The program idea stemmed from conversations Sheikh has had with patients, as well as from all the times she can count that she *did not* have a chance to discuss trials with her patients. She elaborated that patients consistently rate their own doctors as their most trusted source of health information, but most physicians do not have sufficient time or resources to discuss clinical trials with patients (Hesse et al., 2010). "Project PURPLE allows patients to learn about clinical trials through interactive content using custom-built physician avatars modeled after patients' real-life treating physicians," she added. The tool will have an avatar for Sheikh herself, as well as for her colleague, Dr. Alfredo Rivadeneira, who is providing his voice for his avatar, which will have English and Spanish language options.

Creating a Health-Literate Clinical Trials Environment

Sheikh described some of the work done at UNC's clinical trials program at the Thurston Arthritis Research Center, including their five major efforts to create health-literate clinical trials environments, and adopting universal precautions (see Box 4-2). She closed her talk by saying that health literacy in clinical trials is in a dynamic state influenced by how well we deliver information that matches patients' abilities, needs, and preferences, and that informed decisions equal empowered patients.

> **BOX 4-2**
> **Strategies for Creating a Health-Literate Clinical Trials Environment**
>
> - **Educating All Patients About Clinical Trials**
>   o Address implicit biases
>   o Advocate for consideration of participation, rather than participation
>   o Clarify to patients that a doctor–patient relationship will remain unaffected regardless of their decision to participate in a clinical trial
>   o Offer patients resources to help them make informed decisions
> - **Educating Providers About Clinical Trials**
>   o Educate rheumatologists, as well as primary care physicians, subspecialists, and health care teams
> - **Targeted Outreach**
>   o Target patients as well as their health care providers and teams
> - **Communication**
>   o Communicate with all physicians who care for patients enrolled in the trial
>   o Have patients sign a release of information so the clinical trial team can share information about study visits with patients' providers
> - **Expanding Organizational Health Literacy**
>   o Develop a multistep informed consent process (e.g., mail and e-mail copies, follow-up phone calls, and conversation)
>   o Develop customizable template of frequently asked questions for patients
>   o Train teach-back to research personnel as well as to patients
>   o Develop consent forms and supplementary information in languages other than English
>
> SOURCE: Adapted from a presentation by Saira Z. Sheikh at the workshop Health Literacy in Clinical Trials: Practice and Impact on April 11, 2019.

DISCUSSION

Avatars and Technology

Pettit Nassi began the discussion by asking Sheikh about the development of a custom avatar based on a patient's actual physician, and whether she worried if it would ever replace her. Sheikh answered that the idea came from the experience of wanting to have conversations with patients about clinical trials but not always having time. She added that it also enables many more opportunities to provide patient education regarding clinical trials. She continued,

> What tools can we develop so that, while patients are waiting for their appointment and if their doctors are potentially running behind schedule,

patients could be using their time efficiently? In this climate where there are so many burdens and demands on all of us—patients, physicians, other health care providers—we really have to come up with ways that technology can facilitate the things we want to do but are not able to.

The avatar is not meant to replace her, she added, but to provide background knowledge and information and to continue the conversation she had started with her patients.

McCormack added that avatars delivering general information to patients will allow physicians to focus on conversations that are tailored to the patient, and they are also an easy signal to patients that the physician is supportive of the trial.

Spears said that she appreciated the idea that health literacy is not only understanding and appreciation, but also reasoning and the ability to make a choice about participating. She asked if McCormack had found that the method of communication could make a difference in whether a participant felt empowered to make a choice.

McCormack replied that the notion of reasoning through the decision to participate in a clinical trial is very important to her because of its effects on retention.

> If someone doesn't reason through that in advance, when they get to the fact that they have to have blood drawn, or go to the doctor's office, or something else that affects their daily life, that's where we may see them sign a consent form but quit the trial shortly after, because they haven't thought through the implications.
>
> I think the measurement of impact of the work we're doing in health literacy is critical. I know that the field has developed a number of different measures over the years and I think we need to be doing the same thing here, assessing interventions to increase and improve informed consent.

Trudeau added that he liked the avatars and decisional tools, and wondered if the panelists had begun thinking about the scalability of the tools in sites that are not as well funded, and how they would like to see the tools evolve over time. McCormack replied that she and her team have been building a library of assets that will have generalizable content along with tailored elements to certain trials that might have unique avatars or might be a certain specific medication. With the library, she said, there will be a long-term path for efficiency and utility.

Sheikh reiterated that one of the strengths of the tools she and her team have been developing is that, although they may be disease specific, they are clinical trial agnostic. "So you could take it to clinical trials across disease states," she said. "Whenever you develop materials like this, it's always more cost-effective because you can adapt it easily without a lot of work."

Empowered Patients

Jennifer Dillaha from the Arkansas Department of Health asked the panelists to speak more about their experiences with patients and the measurability of "empowered patients." She also asked what defined empowered patients in their experiences.

Arnold responded that empowered patients should first and foremost know that they can withdraw at any time from a trial, and that it is not going to affect the way their provider treats them. McCormack added that, because information is power, patients having access to information helps them make an informed decision, which is one aspect of empowerment.

As an investigator, Sheikh said, she thinks patients that are engaged and empowered are more likely to be retained in studies. Many of her patients are engaged throughout the whole process, she said, and remain as partners even after the clinical trial concludes. "I find that incredibly satisfying," she added.

Nicole Holland from the Tufts University School of Dental Medicine asked if the panelists could elaborate on exactly how they culturally tailor materials for trials. Sheikh replied that when she was developing materials for MIMICT, the patient-input panel reinforced that the faces in the brochures and online guides need to reflect the people that look like them. "It's been an important piece of material development, making sure they reflect the participants." It is not only about the idea of "this person looks like me," she added, but you will not know what cultural or family beliefs might inform someone's decision about participating in a clinical trial unless you ask them. Because of this, it is very important to have ongoing patient input, especially patients from the communities of those participating in trials, she said.

Arnold agreed, saying that all of the photos in materials that they develop are of patients who want to be in the picture. She confirmed that people want to see someone who looks like them but also that they do not want to feel like their group is singled out as representing a disease. Everyone is different, she concluded, which is why it is so important to have focus groups and test your materials.

Collyar said that although it is not "one size fits all," it is important to find out which methods are generalizable. She noted that literacy levels are "just the tip of the iceberg" and that it is important to confirm understanding through the use of tools such as teach-back. Sheikh responded that she agreed and believes that there is a lot of work being done that could be more synergistic and cost-effective because, although the details differ, in many ways the patient experience is similar. She added that convenings such as the workshop provide an opportunity to ask how all of these efforts can be brought together to make this a synergistic process for everybody involved.

McCormack added that perhaps this is an opportunity for members of the roundtable and others in the room to call on funders to accelerate and coordinate their efforts to share information and lessons learned across agencies and organizations. If funding agencies were to use their power to require patient-centered approaches and measuring patient understanding then that would make a big difference, she said. "The [revision to the] Common Rule is a great step forward, but [if] we're not implementing it and funders are not requiring it then we're not going to have progress in this area," she concluded.

Arnold concluded by noting that funders have also shortened their timelines for studies, which allows less time for focus groups and stakeholder engagement. She said that results in some tension for researchers who are trying to develop communications tools and plans but also have to enroll patients quickly.

REFERENCES

Appelbaum, P. S. 2008. MacArthur competence assessment tool for clinical research (MAC-CAT-CR). In *Encyclopedia of psychology and law*. Vol. 1, edited by B. L. Cutler. Thousand Oaks, CA: Sage Publications. P. 464. http://dx.doi.org/10.4135/9781412959537.n178.

Arnold, C. L., A. Rademaker, M. V. Bocchini, P. F. Bass, C. Reynolds, and T. C. Davis. 2009. Rural patients' knowledge, attitude, and behavior about initial and repeat mammography. *American Federation for Medical Research 2009 Southern Regional Meeting Abstracts*. https://afmr.org/abstracts/2009/SR2009_abstracts/335.cgi (accessed January 13, 2020).

Arnold, C. L., A. Rademaker, M. S. Wolf, D. Liu, J. Hancock, and T. C. Davis. 2016a. Third annual fecal occult blood testing in community health clinics. *American Journal of Health Behavior* 40(3):302–309. https://doi.org/10.5993/AJHB.40.3.2.

Arnold, C. L., A. Rademaker, M. S. Wolf, D. Liu, G. Lucas, J. Hancock, and T. C. Davis. 2016b. Final results of a 3-year literacy-informed intervention to promote annual fecal occult blood test screening. *Journal of Community Health* 41(4):724–731. https://doi.org/10.1007/s10900-015-0146-6.

Arnold, C. L., A. Rademaker, D. Liu, and T. C. Davis. 2017. Changes in colorectal cancer screening knowledge, behavior, beliefs, self-efficacy, and barriers among community health clinic patients after a health literacy intervention. *Journal of Community Medicine and Health Education* 7(1):497. doi: 10.4172/2161-0711.1000497.

Arnold, C. L., A. W. Rademaker, J. D. Morris, L. A. Ferguson, G. Wiltz, and T. C. Davis. 2019. Follow-up approaches to a health literacy intervention to increase colorectal cancer screening in rural community clinics: A randomized controlled trial. *Cancer* 125(20):3615–3622. https://doi.org/10.1002/cncr.32398.

Beskow, L. M., L. Lin, C. B. Dombeck, E. Gao, and K. P. Weinfurt. 2017. Improving biobank consent comprehension: A national randomized survey to assess the effect of a simplified form and review/retest intervention. *Genetics in Medicine* 19(5):505–512. https://doi.org/10.1038/gim.2016.157.

Brach, C. 2019. Making informed consent an informed choice. *Health Affairs Blog*, April 4, 2019. https://www.healthaffairs.org/do/10.1377/hblog20190403.965852/full (accessed January 13, 2020).

Brown, R. F., D. L. Cadet, R. H. Houlihan, M. D. Thomson, E. C. Pratt, A. Sullivan, and L. A. Siminoff. 2013. Perceptions of participation in a phase I, II, or III clinical trial among African American patients with cancer: What do refusers say? *Journal of Oncology Practice* 9(6):287–293. doi: 10.1200/JOP.2013.001039.

Coakley, M., E. O. Fadiran, L. J. Parrish, R. A. Griffith, E. Weiss, and C. Carter. 2012. Dialogues on diversifying clinical trials: Successful strategies for engaging women and minorities in clinical trials. *Journal of Women's Health (Larchmont)* 21(7):713–716. https://dx.doi.org/10.1089%2Fjwh.2012.3733.

CTTI (Clinical Trials Transformation Initiative). 2019a. *CTTI recommendations: Informed consent*. https://www.ctti-clinicaltrials.org/files/ctti-informedconsent-recs.pdf (accessed January 13, 2020).

CTTI. 2019b. *Engaging patients and sites*. https://www.ctti-clinicaltrials.org/projects/engaging-patients-and-sites (accessed January 13, 2020).

Davis, T., C. Arnold, A. Rademaker, C. Bennett, S. Bailey, D. Platt, C. Reynolds, D. Liu, E. Carias, P. Bass, and M. Wolf. 2013. Improving colon cancer screening in community clinics. *Cancer* 119(21):3879–3886. https://doi.org/10.1002/cncr.28272.

Davis, T. C., C. L. Arnold, C. L. Bennett, M. S. Wolf, C. Reynolds, D. Liu, and A. Rademaker. 2014a. Strategies to improve repeat fecal occult blood testing cancer screening. *Cancer Epidemiology, Biomarkers & Prevention* 23(1):134–143. doi: 10.1158/1055-9965.

Davis, T. C., A. Rademaker, C. L. Bennett, M. S. Wolf, E. Carias, C. Reynolds, D. Liu, and C. L. Arnold. 2014b. Improving mammography screening among the medically underserved. *Journal of General Internal Medicine* 29(4):628–635. https://doi.org/10.1007/s11606-013-2743-3.

Davis, T. C., C. L. Arnold, C. L. Bennett, M. S. Wolf, D. Liu, and A. Rademaker. 2015a. Sustaining mammography screening among the medically underserved: A follow-up evaluation. *Journal of Women's Health (Larchmont)* 24(4):291–298. doi: 10.1089/jwh.2014.4967.

Davis, T. C., C. L. Arnold, M. S. Wolf, C. L. Bennett, D. Liu, and A. Rademaker. 2015b. Joint breast and colorectal cancer screenings in medically underserved women. *Journal of Community and Supportive Oncology* 13(2):47–54. doi: 10.12788/jcso.0108.

Davis, T. C., A. Rademaker, J. Morris, L. A. Ferguson, G. Wiltz, and C. L. Arnold. 2019. Repeat annual colorectal cancer screening in rural community clinics: A randomized clinical trial to evaluate outreach strategies to sustain screening. *The Journal of Rural Health*. https://doi.org/10.1111/jrh.12399.

FDA (U.S. Food and Drug Administration). 2016. *Use of electronic informed consent—Questions and answers: Guidance for institutional review boards, investigators, and sponsors*. https://www.fda.gov/media/116850/download (accessed January 13, 2020).

Grady, C., S. R. Commings, M. C. Rowbotham, M. V. McConnell, E. A. Ashley, and G. Kang. 2017. Informed consent. *New England Journal of Medicine* 376(9):856–867. doi: 10.1056/NEJMra1603773.

Hesse, B. W., R. P. Moser, and L. J. Rutten. 2010. Surveys of physicians and electronic health information. *The New England Journal of Medicine* 362(9):859–860. doi: 10.1056/NEJMc0909595.

HRSA (Health Resources and Services Administration). 2019. *HRSA health center program fact sheet*. https://bphc.hrsa.gov/sites/default/files/bphc/about/healthcenterfactsheet.pdf (accessed January 13, 2020).

Kim, E. J., and S. H. Kim. 2015. Simplification improves understanding of informed consent information in clinical trials regardless of health literacy level. *Clinical Trials* 12(3):232–236. https://doi.org/10.1177/1740774515571139.

NIH (National Institutes of Health). 2016. *The need for awareness of clinical research*. https://www.nih.gov/health-information/nih-clinical-research-trials-you/need-awareness-clinical-research (accessed January 13, 2020).

NLM (National Library of Medicine). 2019. *Map of all studies on clinicaltrials.gov*. https://clinicaltrials.gov/ct2/search/map (accessed January 13, 2020).

Perrin, A., and E. Turner. 2019. Smartphones help blacks, Hispanics bridge some—but not all—digital gaps with whites. *Pew Research Center, Facttank News in the Numbers*, August 20, 2019. https://www.pewresearch.org/fact-tank/2019/08/20/smartphones-help-blacks-hispanics-bridge-some-but-not-all-digital-gaps-with-whites (accessed January 13, 2020).

Stacey, D., F. Légaré, K. Lewis, M. J. Barry, C. L. Bennett, K. B. Eden, M. Holmes-Rovner, H. Llewellyn-Thomas, A. Lyddiatt, R. Thomson, and L. Trevena. 2017. Decision aids for people facing health treatment or screening decisions. *Cochrane Database of Systematic Reviews* (4):CD001431. https://doi.org/10.1002/14651858.CD001431.pub5.

UN (United Nations). 2013. Deputy UN chief calls for urgent action to tackle global sanitation crisis. *UN News*. https://news.un.org/en/story/2013/03/435102-deputy-un-chief-calls-urgent-action-tackle-global-sanitation-crisis#.UUwW_VrIxZ8 (accessed January 13, 2020).

Vangeepuram, N., V. Mayer, K. Fei, E. Hanlen-Rosado, C. Andrade, S. Wright, and C. Horowitz. 2018. Smartphone ownership and perspectives on health apps among a vulnerable population in East Harlem, New York. *mHealth* 4:31. doi: 10.21037/mhealth.2018.07.02.

5

Designing Clinical Trials with Health Literacy Best Practices

The final workshop panel explored what the future holds for incorporating health literacy into clinical trials from the beginning of the process. Terry C. Davis, professor of medicine and pediatrics at the Louisiana State University Health Sciences Center, moderated the discussion. Each panelist spoke for 5 minutes, giving her insights on the previous presentations and discussions as well as looking ahead. Davis then posed questions and facilitated a discussion with the audience. The panelists were Emma Andrews, senior director in U.S./Global Medical Affairs at Pfizer Biopharmaceutical Group; Monika Mitra, Nancy Lurie Marks Associate Professor of Disability Policy, Lurie Institute for Disability Policy at Brandeis University; Jovonni R. Spinner, senior public health advisor and co-lead for the Outreach and Communications Program at the U.S. Food and Drug Administration's (FDA's) Office of Minority Health and Health Equity (OMHHE); and Rebecca J. Williams, acting director of ClinicalTrials.gov at the National Center for Biotechnology Information of the National Library of Medicine (NLM) at the National Institutes of Health.

PRESENTATIONS

Emma Andrews, Senior Director, U.S./Global Medical Affairs, Pfizer Biopharmaceutical Group

Andrews began by noting that her remarks represented her own views and not those of Pfizer. She continued by saying that she is passionate about health literacy and that she and her colleagues work throughout her organization with the goal of bringing breakthrough medicines that can positively impact people's lives to market. Andrews emphasized that new medicines could not be brought to the market without clinical trials.

Andrews noted, however, that clinical trials could not happen without patients, health care professionals, clinical research investigators, and many others. She said that she would like to expand that list to include, for example, community organizers, teachers, and faith-based leaders. Andrews said that everyone in the community needs to know about clinical trials because there are still a number of myths and misperceptions among people outside of the health care system. She believes that can change through health literacy and clear communication. She also reasserted that health literacy is not about making sure information is communicated in "lay" terms, because everyone could be considered a layperson depending on the topic. Health literacy is achieved by aligning the complexity of health information with the capacity of the intended audience.

Andrews said that, in her opinion, one important area for the future of health literacy in clinical trials is the informed consent process. She likened the process to going to a new restaurant where the food is unfamiliar. The chef may say, "This is an amazing dish," but upon tasting it a person may not like it. According to Andrews, the informed consent process is similar because patients are being told what the clinical trial experience is like but cannot know for sure until they are enrolled in the trial. Andrews hopes that health literacy practices and improved technology developed with health literacy in mind (e.g., virtual reality headsets) can help people better understand what to expect from a clinical trial and therefore increase the number of people who stay in trials after enrollment.

Monika Mitra, Nancy Lurie Marks Associate Professor of Disability Policy, Lurie Institute for Disability Policy, Brandeis University

Mitra began by saying that she has never conducted a clinical trial and is not a patient advocate. Her expertise is in disability policy and, she said, her purpose at the workshop was to speak about inclusion of people with disabilities (PWD) in clinical trials. Specifically, Mitra asked, how can we use the principles of health literacy to inform our research designs so that we can include PWD more effectively?

According to Mitra, there are approximately 54 million people in the United States with a disability, and they are a diverse group with different levels of functioning and different levels of need. Mitra said they are also a group more likely to have more complex health conditions and chronic conditions in addition to their disabling conditions. She said that as a group, PWD are potentially the greatest beneficiaries of clinical trials and health services research. They represent about one-quarter of health expenditures in the United States and face significant health, social, and economic disparities. Finally, Mitra noted, they are traditionally marginalized and underrepresented but, in most research and policy settings, they are not recognized as a group that faces disparities. This exclusion also applies to clinical trials research and it occurs because of both explicit and implicit barriers.

Due to strict inclusion and exclusion criteria, Mitra said, clinical trials have traditionally favored healthy, young, nondisabled Caucasians. According to Mitra, clinical trials exclude about 59 percent of the U.S. population because of these inclusion and exclusion criteria. A considerable number in this group are children and adults with disabilities. Mitra referenced a 2014 study by Feldman and colleagues that reviewed 300 randomized controlled clinical trials and looked specifically at the inclusion of people with intellectual disabilities. They found that, out of the 300 studies, only 6 (2 percent) explicitly included people with intellectual disabilities. They also found that 15 percent explicitly excluded people with intellectual disabilities because of explicit barriers. Mitra asked, "What about trials between the 2 percent that were inclusive and the 15 percent that were exclusive, and what are the implicit barriers between the two margins?"

Feldman and colleagues found that 90 percent of the studies that did not mention people with intellectual disabilities in the inclusion/exclusion criteria were designed in a way that excluded people with these disabilities, said Mitra. These implicit barriers included a lack of community engagement, inaccessible materials and information during recruitment, inadequate representation of PWD, and lack of knowledge and disability competence within the research community (Feldman et al., 2014). Mitra noted that these are examples of the implicit bias and unfounded beliefs within the research and medical communities about the competence of PWD. Mitra said that this is why it is important both to be aware of health literacy and to have a holistic definition of health literacy.

All of this is compounded by a paucity of research and limited understanding of what health literacy is within the context of PWD, said Mitra. Current health literacy efforts often systematically exclude PWD, according to Mitra, and this exclusion contributes to the ongoing health disparities and inequities among those who are disabled. Mitra explained:

> When framing health literacy in PWD, we should think beyond accessible materials. We should think beyond inclusion and exclusion criteria … we should think about the design and implementation of the studies. We should think of the systemic barriers to communication and the facilitation of access and the meaningful engagement of disabled communities. We should also think about understanding the sociocultural context within which health literacy is experienced within the disability community. And

this framing of health literacy is critical for PWD and for other marginalized communities. It is especially important for PWD given the incredible mistrust between PWD and the medical community.

Mitra went on to explain the concept of universal research design, described by Williams and Moore (2011, p. 1), which "promote[s] routine inclusion of persons with disabilities in mainstream biomedical studies, without the need for adaptation or specialized design." She explained that "universal design" was later expanded by Rios and colleagues (2016) into "accessible research design," which sought to broaden the idea of accessible research by considering universal design as one of three levels of implementation, with the second and third being accommodations and modifications, respectively. Agreeing with Rios and colleagues' analysis, Mitra noted that in order to effectively include PWD in clinical trials, the research community needs to move beyond universal design and think of inclusive and accessible research design. This should include the principles of universal design but also accommodation and modification. The research should be inclusive of PWD in all stages of research from study design to recruitment strategies. Most of all, Mitra concluded, it needs to be founded in the principle of the civil rights mantra "nothing about us without us."

Jovonni R. Spinner, Senior Public Health Advisor, Outreach and Communications, Office of Minority Health and Health Equity, U.S. Food and Drug Administration

Spinner began by saying that she would be speaking about the perspective of FDA. This perspective, she said, is that the work of improving health literacy in clinical trials starts before the trial begins. Her mission in the OMHHE is to do this by raising awareness about why diversity in clinical trials is necessary. The mission of the OMHHE, according to Spinner, is to create a world where health equity is a reality for everyone, and a key component of health equity is health literacy.

The OMHHE is interested in promoting better informed decision making about FDA-regulated products, said Spinner. Patients should be involved in every stage of the clinical trials process. Spinner said that the OMHHE wants to make sure that racial and ethnic minorities; veterans; youth; lesbian, gay, bisexual, transgender, or queer individuals; and individuals with limited English proficiency and low health literacy have the health information they need in a form they can access and understand. This allows them to make decisions not just about their own health but for their loved ones as well. Improving health literacy among these populations is critically important to reducing health disparities because low health literacy does have an impact on a person's ability to make decisions about their health, Spinner added. This can range from knowing how to read a medication label, to knowing how to check one's glucose, to understanding what that number means. For issues relating to informed consent, Spinner cited some of the questions:

- Do they know that they are eligible for the trial?
- Do they understand what the inclusion and exclusion criteria mean?
- Do they understand the documentation that has been given to them?

As a result, Spinner said, the OMHHE has a very specific focus on making sure that they are creating culturally and linguistically tailored clinical trial health education resources that are written in plain language at all literacy levels so that everyone can understand. Low health literacy cuts across all levels of education and income; even the savviest person can have low health literacy.

Spinner said that the way the OMHHE prepares people at all levels of health literacy is first by working with stakeholders. This allows the OMHHE to understand where they can improve and whether they have adequately conveyed the appropriate message. The OMHHE does message testing with panels of consumers, Spinner added, asking whether the graphics are appropriate and if the information is clear and easy to understand.

With regard specifically to clinical trials, Spinner leads the Diversity in Clinical Trials Initiative, a multimedia campaign to raise awareness about the importance of minority representation in clinical trials. One of the goals of the campaign, Spinner said, is to dispel some of the myths that exist in racial and ethnic minority communities about clinical trials and to introduce positive messages about clinical trials. The initiative addresses myths such as that a person has to be sick to participate in a clinical trial, said Spinner, adding, "Many people think that a clinical trial is a last resort measure." The initiative also lets people know that research participation is voluntary and that participants can leave at any time without penalty. Spinner said that the initiative also addresses some historical abuses experienced by racial and ethnic minority groups.

According to Spinner, the initiative has produced nine public service announcements (PSAs) so far. The first six feature an African American woman who is an FDA patient representative living with sickle cell disease. Other PSAs and videos feature Spanish speakers, veterans, and other representatives of different populations. It is important to make sure that people see themselves in the material, said Spinner. The initiative is also producing podcasts, social media posts, blogs, newsletters, and a communications tool kit, as well as a number of print materials. Spinner noted that the diversity of materials is important for health literacy because information should be presented in a variety of ways. She added,

> We know that our communities need multiple types of information so we have the videos that are reinforced by the fact sheets, that are reinforced by the social media message, that are reinforced by the stakeholder engagement ... we have this multimedia approach to make sure that people can get the messaging in different ways.

Spinner concluded by summarizing the key health literacy strategies of the OMHHE, including

- using plain language and avoiding jargon;
- assessing audience needs; and
- tailoring materials appropriately, including taking care with translating materials.

Finally, Spinner said, it is important to keep the patient at the center of everything they do and to make sure that patients have the information that they need to make decisions about their health.

Rebecca J. Williams, Acting Director, ClinicalTrials.gov,
National Center for Biotechnology Information,
National Library of Medicine, National Institutes of Health

Williams began by saying that in her role at ClinicalTrials.gov she is privileged to sit at the cross-section of the clinical trials enterprise. She noted that the ClinicalTrials.gov website is intended to serve multiple purposes. First, to provide accountability for the way research is conducted and reported but also to be a resource for people who want to find trials and determine eligibility. Having multiple purposes brings tension, Williams added, and dealing with that is part of looking to the future of health literacy in clinical trials.

In order to talk about the future, Williams said, she would need to talk about the past a little. One of the things that they were asked to consider at ClinicalTrials.gov as part of the rulemaking process for the FDA Amendments Act of 2007 (which expanded which trials are required to be reported and added the requirement that investigators had to submit results) was whether the results had to be accompanied by a narrative summary intended for a general audience. Part of this, Williams noted, was determining whether ClinicalTrials.gov could ensure that the summaries were not promotional or misleading, so her office sought public comment on whether the summaries should be included in the ClinicalTrials.gov database.

According to Williams, her office was particularly concerned about the criterion of ensuring that the summaries are easy to read and not promotional or misleading. They receive 600 new trial registrations every week and post 120 new results records every week, Williams said, so there is no way that staff can have a systematic process for validating information. It is a challenge to ensure that such a massive amount of information is meeting the public's needs and is independent of bias. According to Williams, they did not receive many comments on methods that could resolve the issue so they decided to defer the decision on posting summaries for the public until they could find a way to ensure the quality of the information. But as this process was being considered, they realized that informed consent documents are intended for non-experts and are reviewed by an oversight body. Williams stated that as a first step they could post informed consent documents publicly on ClinicalTrials.gov to accompany the study record. In addition, when the Common Rule revisions came out, it became a requirement to post the informed consent document if the study was funded by a federal agency and covered by the Common Rule. Now there is a trove of informed consent documents available online, said Williams, and this is an opportunity to evaluate those documents and identify best practices.

Another practice that came out of the rulemaking process, said Williams, is that ClinicalTrials.gov now requires, along with the results information that is being posted, that the full protocol document and statistical analysis be reported to allow for the evaluation of the results. It has also been clarified that when the registration is posted, a brief summary that explains what the trial is about must be posted and written in plain language for a general audience, although Williams noted that guidance has not yet been issued on best practices for writing this content. She added that the registration information at ClinicalTrials.gov is meant to be a representation of the information that is in the protocol document itself, a summary of the information that is considered the most important from the study.

When protocol documents were created, Williams said, no one envisioned that they would become a source of public information about the trial. So the way the protocol document is used has been transformed but the way the documents are written and crafted has not yet been transformed. Williams said she believes there is an opportunity to rethink the protocol document and how it can serve not just the study team but also the general public. Williams also noted that a couple of years ago ClinicalTrials.gov had done an evaluation on their website that included all of their different audiences: patients, researchers, health care providers, etc. They found that even the most frequent and advanced users did not fully understand everything they could do or get from the website. Some parts of the website were reworked to respond to this evaluation and, as a part of that, the decision was made to prioritize the needs of the patient in revising the content. What they found, Williams reported, was that by prioritizing patients, the needs of other users were not compromised. In fact, she said, the opposite was true, and the revisions seemed to better support all of their users.

DISCUSSION

Improving Stakeholder Involvement

The first questions from Davis were "How can we do a better job of involving stakeholders? How can we do a better job of identifying who needs to be informed and when and how to inform them?"

Spinner began by noting that the term "stakeholder" is broad and the concept should also be broad. She noted that often people work in silos and do not know who else is working in their space and that it is also beneficial to look for nontraditional partners. For example, she suggested, education, housing, and transportation can all have important impacts on whether people participate in clinical trials. Taking the specific example of transportation, she asked,

> How does the person get to the clinical trial site? Is their neighborhood safe enough for them to get to public transportation? Do they have access to their own car? When you are thinking about a person embarking on a clinical trial you need to make sure that all of the other areas of their life are intact ... you don't want their health to fall at the bottom [of the list] because there is a more pressing issue.

The different sectors need to work together, Spinner concluded, so it is important to bring everyone to the table to have this conversation.

Davis then asked, "In developing a clinical trial, how many people outside of the trial need to be involved? How wide do you cast the net?"

Andrews answered that in the field of pharma, they start with an unmet medical need. Once that need is identified, they determine who the patients are, where they live, and how they relate to their communities. After that, she continued, colleagues may work with patient advocacy organizations that will know that patient population and know who the influencers are within that community, such as faith-based leaders and educators. Colleagues ensure that insights from the patient advocacy organizations are shared with the scientists. Andrews concluded by saying that she would challenge health care professionals to think about where patients live and what their communities are like.

Mitra answered that she is currently conducting research on the perinatal health of women who are deaf and hard of hearing. On this study, there are investigators, research staff, and advisory board members who are deaf and hard of hearing, and they have also involved the National Association of the Deaf. In another research study on women with physical disabilities, Mitra said, two of her co-investigators are women with physical disabilities. It is critically important, she noted, to involve people that represent or understand the experiences of those involved in the study, she said.

Williams noted that a challenge of talking about clinical trials is that everyone assumes they are all equal, which is not the case. She added that it is important to determine the individual preferences and assumptions of participants to help them understand whether a trial is right for them.

Balancing Patient, Community, and Funding Needs for Trials

Davis then asked how investigators can balance the needs of patients and communities with the requirements of the funders of clinical trials.

Williams answered that, often, lack of resources is used as an excuse for not being inclusive or taking health literacy into account. She said that that approach should be flipped; the question should ask what resources are necessary to conduct a high-quality trial, and the answer should determine the design, not the other way around. Mitra noted that it is also necessary to "bake it in"; if funders require the involvement of communities, representation, and health literacy then it will happen.

Davis asked about visual images and messaging and how an investigator can know what is appropriate. Andrews answered that investigators must test the materials they are going to use because no matter how carefully the message has been crafted it could miss the mark in terms of messaging. Spinner echoed this comment, saying that testing the message is vitally important. Mitra added that just having pictures of minorities or PWD is tokenism, and inclusion cannot begin and end with pictures in a brochure. Spinner also added that sometimes it is best not to use people but rather graphics that animate a process; it is important to consider the context. Davis followed up by noting that one of the more powerful examples of this she had seen was a video explaining colonoscopies to children that used a teddy bear instead of a child.

Looking Ahead: Potential Key Changes

Davis then asked the panelists, "If there is one thing that you could change, what are some things that you think are key?"

Andrews said that for her it is getting the message out that the stakeholders are not just physicians and clinical investigators, and that we need to do a better job of educating people about clinical trials. Mitra answered that she thought it was important to build trust and to look at who is not at the table and work for inclusion. Spinner's answer was that she would like scientists and researchers to look at their terminology and stop using jargon and to be creative about how they are getting information out to participants. Finally, Williams answered that she would want researchers to focus on how they intend to communicate from the very beginning of the trial design and to prepare people to receive that information rather than thinking about it as an accessory. She continued by saying that people rely on a single document (the protocol document) to communicate about a specific trial, but right now that document is not meeting people's needs.

Christopher R. Trudeau from the University of Arkansas School of Law asked about the user statistics for ClinicalTrials.gov and whether researchers have been mining the data on the website to improve the process or how they do things. Williams answered that it is used by a wide variety of individuals. In general, she said, about half of their users could be categorized as patients and the public, and the other half as researchers, health care providers, and information professionals like librarians. She added that they do have some patient advocacy organizations that help people navigate the site or their own customized sites and find disease-specific trials and information, which is targeted assistance that the NLM cannot provide. By making the data available, Williams continued, they are helping people to use it in ways that work for them.

Jennifer Dillaha from the Arkansas Department of Health commented that she remembered a study from a number of years ago that found that patients' adherence to HIV medications was strongly predicted by whether they believed the workers at the clinic cared about them. She wondered if adhering to health literacy principles would better communicate to patients that they are cared for. Vanessa Simonds from the University of Montana wondered how researchers and investigators could be held accountable for using health literacy best practices, especially if they do not have a background in health literacy or health communication. Williams noted that this was an important question but she did not know the answer, saying that there should definitely be a discussion around what kind of competencies investigators and researchers should have.

Nicole Holland from the Tufts University School of Dental Medicine asked how researchers can address historical abuses by the research community toward minority communities. Spinner answered that this "dark history" is one of the things they are trying to address with the clinical trials initiative. However, she said, as time passes they have found that it becomes less and less of an issue and that mostly people in underserved communities are not participating in clinical trials because they are not asked. She added that it is important to engage the "gatekeepers of the community" (e.g., faith-based leaders) to start building trust. Mitra noted that she has found that for PWD, the way they interact with clinicians is critically important and if they feel stigmatized or disrespected it becomes a cumulative burden. Andrews responded that, for her, transparency and authenticity are key. It is not just about enrolling people in a trial but sharing the results with them and getting feedback on what went well and how things could have been better. Davis summarized that what she was hearing from everyone was that trust is key and the researchers need to be trustworthy, especially for minority communities.

Pettit Nassi commented that there is currently a moratorium against biospecimen collection that began with the Navajo Nation and went to the Cherokee Nation and is now essentially nationwide for American Indians and Alaska Natives (AIs/ANs). She said that this is a challenge because there are very few from the AI/AN population who are enrolled in clinical trials. It does not matter how trustworthy a researcher is, she said, because historically, native populations' relationship with the federal government has been a challenge. Pettit Nassi said that when we talk about transparency and authenticity, we need to remember that there are still areas—not just AI/AN communities but also small, rural church communities—that have similar challenges, who do not trust the research community. Because of this, a whole population is left behind, she said, adding, "Are the people who make those decisions listening and finding answers to [this problem]?"

Collyar followed up by saying that one thing that could be recommended is that a communication plan must be part of protocol development. She added that there are communication models that are not that difficult to implement and if researchers start to think about communication as a necessary part of developing the plan it would be a fundamental switch.

Duhig asked Williams if there is an opportunity for ClinicalTrials.gov to make a communication plan a requirement or recommend it. He added that smart regulation and requirements like that can have an impact.

Williams answered that she thinks ClinicalTrials.gov might be too late in the process to influence that because people come to them when they have already developed the protocol. However, she said, she does think there are ways to incentivize particular goals, such as requiring certain elements in the document. Andrews responded that she wanted to play devil's advocate by suggesting that because protocol documents are not intended for patients and the public maybe they should not be the documents relied on for communication purposes. She posited that perhaps a different document is necessary, one that is designed for patients and the public. Williams responded that unfortunately the protocol document is the main source document for dissemination currently but that it is definitely worth thinking about whether that should be the case.

Steve Rush from UnitedHealth Group commented that several years ago, United Health Foundation had a grant program that required a communication plan and adherence to health literacy best practices from applicants, so there is some precedent. Barbara Biesecker from RTI International noted a similar experience in her previous work, where she and the study investigator made a commitment in a multiyear study to give the participants a summary of the results every year in easy-to-understand language. They spent time with stakeholders developing a communications plan, and after that, she said, it was not difficult to adhere to the plan. Getting communication right took work, she said, but "there was nothing complicated about it."

REFERENCES

Feldman, M. A., J. Bosett, C. Collet, and P. Burnham-Riosa. 2014. Where are persons with intellectual disabilities in medical research? A survey of published clinical trials. *Journal of Intellectual Disability Research* 58(9):800–809. doi: 10.1111/jir.12091.

Rios, D., S. Magasi, C. Novak, and M. Harniss. 2016. Conducting accessible research: Including people with disabilities in public health, epidemiological, and outcomes studies. *American Journal of Public Health* 106(12):2137–2144. doi: 10.2105/ajph.2016.303448.

Williams, A. S., and S. M. Moore. 2011. Universal design of research: Inclusion of persons with disabilities in mainstream biomedical studies. *Science Translational Medicine* 3(82):82cm12. doi: 10.1126/scitranslmed.3002133.

6

Reflections, Research Directions, and Potential Opportunities for Implementation

RAPPORTEUR PRESENTATIONS

During the first half of the final session of the workshop, participants who had been designated as rapporteurs provided brief summaries of the presentations and discussions that had taken place over the preceding three sessions. The rapporteurs' descriptions of their key takeaways were intended to stimulate discussion during the last reflections session of the workshop. Patty Spears shared her key takeaways from the day as a cancer survivor and a scientific research manager and patient advocate at the University of North Carolina Lineberger Comprehensive Cancer Center, and Consuelo H. Wilkins shared her summary and takeaways as vice president for health equity at the Vanderbilt University Medical Center and associate dean for health equity at Vanderbilt University. Wilkins also shared a brief description of her work as a co-principal investigator for the Recruitment Innovation Center (RIC). A summary of selected points highlighted by each rapporteur is provided in Box 6-1.

Recruitment Innovation Center: Opportunities to Incorporate Health Literacy Principles

Consuelo H. Wilkins, Vice President for Health Equity, Vanderbilt University

In addition to describing her key takeaways, Wilkins shared some challenges and successes she had experienced through her work at the RIC,

BOX 6-1
Highlights from Rapporteur Presentations

During the final session of the workshop, two rapporteurs presented key takeaways of the workshop's previous three sessions. Selected highlights from each of the rapporteur's presentations are presented below.

- Context and words are important for clinician–patient relationships. Terms like "recruitment and retention" or "subject" are not patient-friendly terms, and can do a disservice to patients. (Spears, Wilkins)
- Investigators need to share information that patients actually want to know, not only information investigators want them to know. (Spears)
- Investigators need to know their audiences, because one size never fits all and never will. Patient engagement is necessary. It is a common perception that it will slow the trial down or cost more, but, in the end, if your trial does not accrue any patients, it is a waste of time and money. (Spears)
- Patients are not homogeneous and neither are experiences of stages of disease. For example, newly diagnosed breast cancer patients have incredibly different experiences and reactions than metastatic patients who have picked up knowledge during their years of treatment. (Spears)
- Incorporating health literacy principles is necessary for clear communication about benefits and risks of participation, returning trial results, and general clinical trial materials. (Wilkins)
- There are elements of health literacy that go well beyond plain language, and many clinical investigators are unfamiliar with these aspects. (Wilkins)
- Timing should be a major consideration for clinical investigators. It is better to give patients the chance to take materials home—to make it the best learning situation for the patient, and not what best fits the clinical care schedule. That could include multiple sessions or follow-up phone calls. (Spears)
- Clinical trial education should be provided to patients when they have been diagnosed with a chronic disease or cancer, regardless of their eligibility status. (Spears, Wilkins)
- Implementing health literacy principles in clinical trials will require a variety of players and resource sharing, as well as patients as partners, network building, and outcome metrics, including patient-centric metrics. (Spears)
- Investigators and their teams need more templates, tools, and resources for improving the informed consent process. (Wilkins)
- Resources and tools to improve health literacy in clinical trials are going to require funds, time, and training. (Wilkins)
- More research is needed to identify potential funders for developing and incorporating new health literacy resources and tools in clinical trials. (Wilkins)
- More work is needed to identify and measure outcomes connected with health literacy principles in clinical trials. (Wilkins)

SOURCE: Adapted from remarks by Patty Spears and Consuelo H. Wilkins at the workshop Health Literacy in Clinical Trials: Practice and Impact on April 11, 2019.

which serves multisite trials and is part of the Trial Innovation Network, a collaborative initiative within the National Institutes of Health Clinical Translational Science Awards program.[1] A major focus of the RIC, she said, is minority recruitment, where "a fair amount of our health-literacy-related work is happening," though she added that "health literacy" is not a frequently used term among RIC teams. One such example was a supplemental online course for clinical investigators and staff, called "Faster Together: Enhancing the Recruitment of Minorities in Clinical Trials," which was developed with input from minority groups. The course shares strategies for recruiting racial and ethnic minorities, she added, including providing culturally tailored materials.[2] Wilkins noted that the course is free and intended to help recruiters improve their minority recruitment, communicate effectively, and build relationships and trust.

The RIC also developed TrialsToday.org from ResearchMatch.org, Wilkins explained, which culls all the information available at Clinical Trials.gov, and provides a user-friendly sorting and filtering process for potential participants to find trials for which they might be eligible. More recently, the RIC translated the website for Spanish speakers. When beginning their process, Wilkins knew that the website would need to be accessible beyond the literal translation of English to Spanish; she recommended that they lower the reading level to fourth grade before they started the translation. "In the United States," she said, "people who are Spanish speaking, and not bilingual, typically have a lower reading level than average. We needed to lower the ResearchMatch website reading level accordingly" (Jacobson et al., 2016). She added that her team would have benefited from guidelines for adapting and translating those materials using health literacy principles. The RIC has recently developed or is currently developing several mobile apps, including MyCAP—participant-centered data capture that can be shared with investigators—and an app for clinicians to share information. Wilkins noted that she looked forward to explicitly embedding health literacy principles into her work with the RIC.

ROUNDTABLE DISCUSSION

During the remainder of the final session, some members of the Roundtable on Health Literacy identified key themes they had observed throughout the course of the day. A summary of selected observations and points made during this discussion can be found in Box 6-2.

---

[1] For more information about the RIC, see https://trialinnovationnetwork.org/recruitment-innovation-center (accessed October 15, 2019).

[2] The course can be viewed at https://trialinnovationnetwork.org/wp-content/uploads/2019/05/Introduction-to-the-course_-Faster-Together-Enhancing-the-Recruitment-of-Minorities-in-Clinical-Trials.mp4 (accessed October 15, 2019).

> **BOX 6-2**
> **Key Observations from Roundtable Members**
>
> During the final session of the workshop, roundtable members offered their key takeaways and highlights from the day. Selected points from each of the roundtable members are presented below.
>
> - Physicians have a unique role in trial recruitment and should be educated regularly about clinical trials available near them or their patients. (Davis, Robinson, Smith)
> - Because community relationships and trust are a crucial component of clinical trial recruitment, increasing the number of physicians from diverse backgrounds, including racial, ethnic, disability, sexual orientation, and socioeconomic backgrounds, is necessary to recruiting and retaining a more diverse range of participants in trials. (McKee, Robinson, Smith)
> - Research teams should inquire about trial participants' limitations or disabilities. When research teams are not aware of participants' limitations or disabilities, it can negatively affect the robustness of the data collected to build an evidence base. (McKee)
> - Patient advocates can serve important roles on research teams by being more likely to mirror participants and by helping to develop informed consent forms and processes or recruitment materials from a patient perspective. (McKee)
> - Simplifying language around clinical trials can demonstrate caring and understanding to research participants. This is key because trials require people to give their bodies and minds to something that requires their full participation. (Rush)
> - Incorporating health literacy principles into clinical trials should not start with recruitment, but rather with the research team understanding the participant community history or context that might affect recruitment down the line. (Holland)
> - Clinical trials could benefit from having health literacy principles embedded within many touchpoints throughout the process. (Holland, Parnell)
> - There is an opportunity for a group or regulatory body to take ownership of embedding health literacy principles in clinical trials. (Holland, Parnell)
> - Without any training or guidance, it can be difficult for investigators to translate informed consent documents into clear, plain language for patients. Embedding and mandating health literacy principles in trial processes like informed consent would offer much needed guidance and clarity to researchers. (Duhig)
> - The evidence base for health literacy improving patient outcomes in clinical trials needs to be developed so that the field can have the credibility of other evidence-based science fields. (Assaf)

- Communication plans tailored to each clinical trial could help embed health literacy principles throughout the trial process. (Davis, Parnell)
- Health literacy empowers patients and drives health equity. (Willis)
- One version of clinical trial engagement, participation, or recruitment is not always appropriate for all participants, even within the same community. (Willis)
- Research teams should take more responsibility to return trial results to participants and recognize the impact that receiving or not receiving those results can have on communities, particularly communities of color. (Shiyanbola, Willis)
- A module-based approach to informed consent is commonly used outside the research consent world, and incorporating it into clinical trials could improve the whole process. (Trudeau)
- Research protocols should be written in plain language. (Trudeau)
- Informed consent goes well beyond the signed document and is perhaps better conceptualized from a perspective that treats it as an educational process that uses health education and community engagement principles. (Simonds)
- It is necessary for research teams to build trust among groups that have been marginalized by or given reason to mistrust the medical community. (Simonds)
- There is a tension between fast-tracking enrollment and building authentic and transparent relationships with patients, and that tension must be reduced to improve the clinical trial process for everyone. (Robinson)
- During recruitment and enrollment, it is important to consider a patient's fit with and readiness for a clinical trial. (Shiyanbola)
- Research teams should treat federally qualified health centers as individual organizations because they serve a variety of geographies, communities, and individuals. (Daus)
- It is good practice for translators to work only on final drafts to provide accessible materials. (Daus)
- Building relationships, developing multimodal materials, developing interventions that make use of new technology, and centering patients are all components of health literacy principles across health and medicine, not just clinical trials. (Harris)

SOURCES: Adapted from remarks by Annlouise R. Assaf, Gem Daus from the Health Resources and Services Administration, Terry C. Davis, Jennifer Dillaha, Jay Duhig, Linda Harris, Nicole Holland, Michael McKee, Terri Ann Parnell from Health Literacy Partners, Lindsey Robinson from the California Dental Association, Steven Rush, Olayinka Shiyanbola, Vanessa Simonds, Lawrence G. Smith, Christopher R. Trudeau, and Earnestine Willis from the Medical College of Wisconsin at the workshop Health Literacy in Clinical Trials: Practice and Impact on April 11, 2019.

Discussion

Smith observed that many barriers to clinical trial recruitment challenges had been identified over the years but was uncertain about how many had truly been addressed. He added

> We don't have a [medical] workforce that reflects minority patients culturally, historically, or racially. Until we do, we are all doing workarounds over the fact that those participants do not have physicians that they trust enough to be referred into trials without constantly fearing that they are going to be either marginalized or abused in the trials.

Smith added that he was curious about whether there would be any change with regard to the numbers of underrepresented physicians, given that the New York University School of Medicine had announced the previous summer that all students would receive full-tuition scholarships for the M.D. program.[3]

Dillaha asked, "How do we flip it so medical science serves people, as opposed to people serving medical science?"

Assaf wondered how to build bridges across the variety of stakeholders invested in improving patient outcomes and helping people live healthier lives by embedding health literacy into clinical trials, and how to include newer technology in such efforts.

Simonds noted that the findings discussed at the workshop should be reflected in Institutional Review Board policies, and those policies should be enforced with tools and incentives to improve the informed consent process.

Harris noted that she appreciated the diversity of speakers and experiences represented at the workshop.

Smith thanked the roundtable staff, workshop planning committee, and speakers, concluding, "This set of presentations was inspiring, informative, provocative, edgy, and convincing. I think it created a discussion that was among the best I've ever seen."

REFERENCE

Jacobson, H. E., L. Hund, and F. Soto Mas. 2016. Predictors of English health literacy among U.S. Hispanic immigrants: The importance of language, bilingualism and sociolinguistic environment. *Literacy and Numeracy Studies* 24(1):43–64. doi: 10.5130/lns.v24i1.4900.

---

[3] For more information about New York University's full-tuition scholarship for medical students, see https://nyulangone.org/news/nyu-school-medicine-offers-full-tuition-scholarships-all-new-current-medical-students (accessed October 15, 2019).

Appendix A

Workshop Agenda

BOX A-1
Workshop Objectives and Questions

The workshop will address the following questions:

- Why are health literacy practices important for clinical trials?
- What is the state of the science for incorporating health literacy practices into the design and execution of clinical trials?
- How can health literacy improve the quality and outcomes of clinical trials?
- What are the challenges and best practices for incorporating health literacy into clinical trials?

THURSDAY, APRIL 11, 2019

7:45–8:15 AM   REGISTRATION

8:30–8:40 AM   WELCOME AND WORKSHOP OVERVIEW
Lawrence G. Smith, Roundtable on Health Literacy

8:40–10:00 AM   SESSION 1: HEALTH LITERACY IS AN ETHICAL IMPERATIVE IN CLINICAL TRIALS

8:40–9:00 AM	**Keynote 1: Why Health Literacy Matters** *Barbara E. Bierer, Multi-Regional Clinical Trials Center of Brigham and Women's Hospital and Harvard*
9:00–9:20 AM	**Keynote 2: How Health Literacy Helps Patients Make Decisions** *Deborah Collyar, Patient Advocates in Research*
9:20–10:00 AM	**Moderated Discussion** *Moderator: Larry G. Smith*
10:00–10:15 AM	**BREAK**
10:15 AM– 12:15 PM	**SESSION 2: EMBEDDING HEALTH LITERACY INTO CLINICAL TRIALS FROM THE BEGINNING OF THE PROCESS TO IMPROVE RECRUITMENT AND RETENTION**
10:15–11:30 AM	**Presentations and Panelist Discussion** *Ebony Boulware, Duke University School of Medicine* *Catina O'Leary, Health Literacy Media* *Alicia Staley, Medidata Solutions* *Christopher R. Trudeau, University of Arkansas Medical School and Bowen School of Law, University of Arkansas at Little Rock* *Moderator: Annlouise R. Assaf, Pfizer Worldwide Medical and Safety*
11:30 AM– 12:15 PM	**Discussion**
12:15–1:15 PM	**BREAK**
1:15–2:45 PM	**SESSION 3: EXPERIENCES IN IMPLEMENTING HEALTH LITERACY IN CLINICAL TRIALS**
1:15–2:00 PM	**Presentations** *Connie Arnold, Louisiana State University Health Sciences Center*

APPENDIX A 89

                Lauren McCormack, Public Health Research,
                    RTI International
                Saira Z. Sheikh, University of North Carolina
                    School of Medicine

2:00–2:45 PM   Moderated Discussion
                Moderator: Phyllis J. Pettit Nassi, Huntsman
                    Cancer Institute

2:45–3:00 PM   **BREAK**

3:00–4:30 PM   **SESSION 4: WHAT DOES THE FUTURE HOLD FOR DESIGNING CLINICAL TRIALS USING HEALTH LITERACY BEST PRACTICES?**

3:00–4:00 PM   Moderated Panel Discussion
                Emma Andrews, Pfizer Biopharmaceuticals Group
                Monika Mitra, Brandeis University
                Jovonni R. Spinner, Office of Minority Health,
                    U.S. Food and Drug Administration
                Rebecca J. Williams, ClinicalTrials.gov
                Moderator: Terry C. Davis, Louisiana State University
                    Health Sciences Center

4:00–4:30 PM   Discussion

4:30–4:50 PM   **SESSION 5: WORKSHOP HIGHLIGHTS**
                Patty Spears, University of North Carolina Lineberger
                    Comprehensive Cancer Center
                Consuelo H. Wilkins, Vanderbilt University
                    Medical Center

4:50–5:30 PM   **SESSION 6: ROUNDTABLE REFLECTIONS ON THE DAY**
                Moderator: Lawrence G. Smith

5:30 PM   **ADJOURN**

Appendix B

Biographical Sketches of Workshop Moderators, Speakers, and Panelists

Emma Andrews, Pharm.D., is the senior director at Pfizer U.S./Global Medical Affairs, Women's Health, with a focus on Pfizer's menopause portfolio. Dr. Andrews joined Pfizer Worldwide Medical and Safety in 1999 and has held different positions with increasing responsibility in operations, research, and strategy, most recently as the regional medical therapeutic area lead of the Diversified Portfolio for Latin America, where she is responsible for developing medical strategies for Latin America and enhancing medical communication between Pfizer and the region's stakeholders. Prior to that role, Dr. Andrews was a director in External Medical Affairs, responsible for engaging with external partners critical to Pfizer's business with the goal of advancing areas of mutual interest. She was also a member of the Clinical Pharmacology team in New York, working in the infectious diseases therapeutic area, where her main focus was on HIV and malaria.

Dr. Andrews is a registered pharmacist in the state of Connecticut and a member of several health professional organizations. Born in Uganda, Dr. Andrews did her secondary education in Cote d'Ivoire and is trilingual, speaking English, French, and Luganda. She is a past president of the Jack and Jill Inc., Bridgeport, Connecticut, chapter, a position she held from May 2010 to May 2012. Dr. Andrews holds a B.S. in pharmacy and a Pharm.D. from the Massachusetts College of Pharmacy.

Connie Arnold, Ph.D., is a professor of medicine and a medical sociologist at Louisiana State University Health Sciences Center–Shreveport and the Feist-Weiller Cancer Center. Dr. Arnold has more than 26 years of experience conducting health literacy research and has 55 publications on health literacy, health communication and behavior, and preventive medicine. She has a productive record of federally funded research on developing and implementing low literacy interventions to improve health outcomes in vulnerable populations. Her wide-ranging work focuses on improving cancer screening in rural federally qualified health centers (FQHCs), self-management of diabetes in safety-net settings, and the use of health coaches to facilitate weight loss for patients using community clinics. Dr. Arnold is the principal investigator (PI) on a 5-year American Cancer Society health literacy intervention to evaluate follow-up strategies to improve regular colorectal screening in rural FQHCs in the state. She is a site PI and health literacy core co-director on a National Institutes of Health Institutional Development Award grant for the Louisiana Clinical and Translational Science Center, an unprecedented collaborative effort among 11 academic institutions in Louisiana. She is also a site PI on a Pennington Biomedical Center Patient-Centered Outcomes Research Institute–funded grant studying the comparative effectiveness of obesity treatment options delivered in primary care settings for underserved populations. Dr. Arnold has extensive experience working to simplify consent forms and patient education documents. She also has experience working with regional safety-net clinics, providers, and patients to develop and test literacy appropriate interventions.

Annlouise R. Assaf, Ph.D., M.S., FAHA, FISPE, is a pharmacoepidemiologist who is the patient health activation expert and global medical impact assessment senior director for Pfizer Worldwide Medical and Safety. In this role, she partners to evolve the science and practice of benefit–risk to inform better outcomes for patients, drug development, and health care decisions. A focus of her work is on quality benefit–risk communication and improving health literacy and patient-centered medication prescription so that patients can make informed, shared decisions about their treatment, as well as use their medications safely and appropriately, and improve value outcomes. Dr. Assaf is also a co-lead on the Health Literacy Working Group at Pfizer.

Dr. Assaf joined Pfizer in 2002 after many years in academic medicine and clinical research at the Brown University Medical School. She received her doctorate from the Roswell Park Cancer Institute in Buffalo, where she focused her research efforts in the fields of cancer and cardiovascular disease epidemiology with a particular focus on diseases that disproportionately affect women and patients with low health literacy.

Dr. Assaf was the co-principal investigator (PI) of the Pawtucket Heart Health Program, a community-based intervention for the prevention of cardiovascular disease, where she specialized in the evaluation of programs aimed at behavior change in low health literacy, low-income, and minority populations.

Dr. Assaf has been the PI or the co-PI for numerous National Institutes of Health clinical trials. She was a PI and Executive Committee member of the Women's Health Initiative (WHI) Clinical Trial and Observational study and ran the largest of the 40 clinical centers of the WHI. She has served in numerous teaching, consulting, and leadership roles nationally and internationally and is currently a professor (adjunct) at the Brown University School of Public Health. She has published more than 100 scientific articles, book chapters, and abstracts.

Barbara E. Bierer, M.D., is a hematologist-oncologist and a professor of medicine at Harvard Medical School and Brigham and Women's Hospital (BWH). Dr. Bierer co-founded and now leads the Multi-Regional Clinical Trials Center of BWH and Harvard (MRCT Center) (www.mrctcenter.org), a collaborative effort to improve standards for the planning and conduct of international clinical trials. The MRCT Center is specifically focusing on health literacy in clinical research. In addition, Dr. Bierer is the director of the Regulatory Foundations, Ethics, and the Law program of Harvard Catalyst, the Harvard Clinical and Translational Science Award, working across the academic spectrum to enable clinical trials. She is the director of regulatory policy for SMART IRB (www.SMARTIRB.org), a national effort to align single-site Institutional Review Board reviews of multisite trials, and she co-founded Vivli (www.Vivli.org), a center for global clinical trial data sharing. From 2003 to 2014, Dr. Bierer served as the senior vice president, research, at BWH. During her tenure, Dr. Bierer founded and served as the executive sponsor of the Brigham Research Institute and the Brigham Innovation Hub (iHub), a focus for entrepreneurship and innovation in health care. She has authored more than 200 publications.

Dr. Bierer has been involved in policy development relating to the oversight of human research protection programs. She has been president of Association for the Accreditation of Human Research Protection Programs, served as chair of the U.S. Department of Health and Human Services' Secretary's Advisory Committee on Human Research Protections, and is currently a board member of Public Responsibility in Medicine and Research, Management Sciences for Health, Vivli, and the Edward P. Evans Foundation. Dr. Bierer received a B.S. from Yale University and an M.D. from Harvard Medical School.

Ebony Boulware, M.D., M.P.H., is a professor of medicine, the chief of the Division of General Internal Medicine in the Department of Medicine, the vice dean for translational science and the associate vice chancellor for translational research in the School of Medicine at Duke University. She received an A.B. from Vassar College, an M.D. from Duke University, and an M.P.H. from the Johns Hopkins Bloomberg School of Public Health.

Dr. Boulware attended medical school at Duke University, followed by residency and 1 year as chief resident in internal medicine at the University of Maryland. She then completed a research fellowship in general internal medicine at Johns Hopkins, where she remained on faculty for more than 10 years. In 2013, she was appointed the chief of the Division of General Internal Medicine in the Duke Department of Medicine. In 2015, she was appointed the director of Duke's Clinical and Translational Science Award. Subsequently, she became the inaugural director of the Duke Clinical and Translational Science Institute.

Dr. Boulware has spent the majority of her scholarly career investigating mechanisms to improve the quality and equity of care and health outcomes for patients and populations with chronic diseases, such as chronic kidney disease and hypertension. Dr. Boulware's research has been funded by numerous organizations, including the National Institutes of Health, the Patient-Centered Outcomes Research Institute, the Health Resources and Services Administration, the Agency for Healthcare Research and Quality, and foundations. She has published more than 120 manuscripts and has mentored numerous students, fellows, and faculty members in clinical research. Dr. Boulware frequently engages community members, patients, their family members, and other stakeholders to develop and implement relevant and sustainable interventions to improve health.

Deborah Collyar is the founder and president of Patient Advocates in Research (PAIR), an international communication network of patient advocates who work with research communities, advocacy organizations, and patients. The network covers multiple diseases, including cancers, rare diseases, and infectious diseases. In her current role, Ms. Collyar educates people about research and shares real patient experiences throughout the research process while helping to translate discoveries into clinical use. Ms. Collyar also founded the Clinical Trial Information Project, which helped cancer patients understand research studies and access open clinical trials, and which prompted the National Cancer Institute (NCI) to redesign its information system.

Ms. Collyar authored an e-book titled *DCIS Dilemmas: Discussions About Ductal Carcinoma in Situ and Research Behind It* and a blog called *One Health of a Life*, in addition to articles on patient advocacy and communication. She is also an editorial board member for the *DIA Global Forum* online monthly magazine, and does reviews for several journals.

Ms. Collyar volunteers with the Alliance for Clinical Trials in Oncology as the vice chair of the Publications Committee, and as a member of the Ethics, Health Outcomes, Experimental Therapeutics, and Patient Advocacy Committees. She was the first patient advocate in the NCI Clinical Trials Network and is a leader in public trial results summaries. She is also a faculty member in the American Association for Cancer Research/American Society of Clinical Oncology Vail Methods in Clinical Research Workshop and the Society for Immunotherapy of Cancer Immunotherapy Winter School.

Terry C. Davis, Ph.D., is a professor of medicine and pediatrics in the Feist Weiller Cancer Center at the Louisiana State University Health Sciences Center in Shreveport, Louisiana. For the past 35 years, she has investigated the impact of patient literacy on health and health care, and she has more than 140 publications related to health communication. Her achievements include the development of the Rapid Estimate of Adult Literacy in Medicine and of user-friendly patient education and provider training materials that are used nationally. Dr. Davis has served on health literacy advisory boards for the American Medical Association and the American College of Physicians as well as on the U.S. Food and Drug Administration's Center for Drug Evaluation and Research. She is a member of the National Academies of Sciences, Engineering, and Medicine's Roundtable on Health Literacy, Healthy People 2020, Health Literacy/Health Communication Section, and she serves on the U.S. Pharmacopeia Convention Expert Panel on Health Literacy. She received the Louisiana Public Health Association's Founders Award for Significant Achievement in Public Health Research. Dr. Davis has a productive record of federally funded research on developing and implementing low literacy interventions to improve the health outcomes of vulnerable populations. Her wide-ranging work focuses on improving cancer screening in rural, federally qualified health centers; the self-management of diabetes in safety net settings; the use of health coaches to facilitate weight loss in community clinics; and improving prescription medication labeling.

Lauren McCormack, Ph.D., M.S.P.H., is the vice president of RTI's Public Health Research Division and an adjunct associate professor at the University of North Carolina (UNC) Gillings School of Global Public Health. Her research bridges the fields of health communication and health policy and involves developing, testing, and evaluating interventions to promote patient-centered care, patient engagement, and informed decision making. An overarching goal of her work is to improve the public's understanding and use of medical evidence in health care decision making. Dr. McCormack is the principal investigator of a 5-year, $9 million pragmatic trial examining the comparative effectiveness of two behavioral interventions focused on opioid use and the management of chronic pain. This study, funded by the Patient-Centered Outcomes Research Institute (PCORI), is a collaboration with Duke University, UNC at Chapel Hill, and Vanderbilt University, and leverages the PCORnet Clinical Data Research Network. She recently completed a study to assist the U.S. Food and Drug Administration (FDA) in enhancing its communications about opioids to both the lay public and health care professionals, and she has provided consultative services to FDA on drug safety messaging. From 2015 to 2018, Dr. McCormack served as chair of PCORI's Clinical Effectiveness and Decision Science Advisory Panel and recently completed a commissioned chapter for the National Academies of Sciences, Engineering, and Medicine on health literacy. She developed a skills-based measure of health literacy and was a guest editor of a series of special issues of the *Journal of Health Communication* focused on health literacy. Dr. McCormack has published more than 60 peer-reviewed manuscripts and multiple book chapters, and she is a frequent presenter at domestic and international conferences.

Monika Mitra, Ph.D., M.A., M.Sc., is the Nancy Lurie Marks Associate Professor of Disability Policy and director of the Lurie Institute for Disability Policy at Brandeis University. She is also adjunct associate professor in the Department of Family Medicine and Community Health at the University of Massachusetts Medical School. Her research examines the health care experiences and health outcomes of people with disabilities, with a particular focus on the sexual and reproductive health of women with disabilities. Her current research revolves around the health needs and barriers to perinatal care among women with disabilities, including women with intellectual and developmental disabilities and deaf and hard-of-hearing women. She is currently co-leading the National Research Center for Parents with Disabilities, with a focus on addressing knowledge gaps regarding the needs of parents with diverse disabilities, and the Community Living Policy Center, aimed at improving policies and practices that advance community living outcomes for people with disabilities. Dr. Mitra is a member of the *Disability and Health Journal* editorial board and of the Advisory Committee of the Academy Health Disability Research Interest Group.

Catina O'Leary, Ph.D., M.S.W., is the president and the chief executive officer of Health Literacy Media (HLM). Accordingly, she oversees HLM's core activities, including the Clearly Communicating Clinical Trials program, and she works to set and maintain the strategic vision for the organization. Dr. O'Leary has steered the organization onto the course of becoming a true partner to a broad spectrum of health care organizations around the world. A primary goal is to empower people with health information they can actually use.

Prior to joining HLM, for more than a decade Dr. O'Leary led research at the Washington University School of Medicine with a focus on connecting people at risk for health conditions such as HIV and other sexually transmitted infections, and with medical and social resources aimed at improving health behaviors, preventing illness, and improving overall health and well-being. During that time, Dr. O'Leary led multisite clinical trials in the United States and internationally. She was actively engaged in every phase of the research process—writing grants to federal agencies and foundations; developing protocols for submission to obtain and maintain Institutional Review Board approval across multiple sites; hiring and training staff for data collection and intervention implementation; and leading data analysis, reporting, and research dissemination.

While at Washington University, Dr. O'Leary was an active member of the Human Research Protection Office's (HRPO's) continuing review committee. Currently, she serves on Washington University's HRPO consent task force, which is focused on adjustments to the university's consent process. She also participates on the Multi-Regional Clinical Trails Center of Brigham and Women's Hospital and Harvard's Health Literacy Workgroup, which is focused on health-literate communication of clinical research information.

Phyllis J. Pettit Nassi, M.S.W., is an Alliance for Clinical Trials in Oncology patient advocate serving on the Patient Advocate, Health Disparities, and Pharmacogenetics and Population Pharmacology Committees; an Advocate in Science member for Susan G. Komen for the Cure; co-chair of the Southwest Region of the Intercultural Cancer Council Network; and a member of the American Association for Cancer Researchers. Enrolled in the Otoe-Missouri tribe, a member of the Cherokee Nation, Ms. Pettit Nassi is the associate director for Research and Science, Special Populations, American Indian Program at the Huntsman Cancer Institute at the University of Utah. Raised on the Navajo, Hopi, and Zuni reservations and experienced in scientific research, outreach, development, and implementation of research projects, Ms. Pettit Nassi is well aware of the need for cultural humility and awareness and works with research teams to understand "how complicated it's going to be to get it right, and how difficult it will be for every researcher working with Native American people if they get it wrong." Formerly a Ph.D. student at the University of Utah's College of Social Work, her focus is on health disparities; the medically underserved of rural and frontier populations; and cancer research education, screening, and early detection. Educating tribal populations about the importance of participating in clinical trials and ensuring their understanding of the future direction of cancer research (e.g., genomics) and data sharing will improve and bring equity to the research table. She has studied cultural and social implications on underserved populations for more than 30 years.

Saira Z. Sheikh, M.D., is an assistant professor of medicine at the University of North Carolina (UNC) at Chapel Hill, the director of the UNC Rheumatology Lupus Clinic, and the director of clinical trials programs at the UNC Thurston Arthritis Research Center. She came to UNC after residency and chief residency in internal medicine at the University of Arizona, and she completed fellowships in rheumatology and allergy immunology at UNC. She is board certified in internal medicine, rheumatology, and allergy and immunology. Her work focuses on answering scientific questions that directly impact the care of patients with lupus and Sjogren's syndrome.

Dr. Sheikh is the principal investigator (PI) on numerous clinical trials evaluating novel therapeutics in lupus. She is leading national initiatives to develop real-world, practical models to improve the education of patients and to change providers' practices to promote inclusion of minority patients in lupus clinical trials, including working with the American College of Rheumatology, funded by the U.S. Department of Health and Human Services' Office of Minority Health. Dr. Sheikh is the co-PI of the Patient Advocates for Lupus Studies program through Lupus Therapeutics, an innovative peer-to-peer educational program, in which patient education is delivered by trained patient advocates who have personal experience with clinical trials.

Dr. Sheikh is interested in using technology-based applications to improve understanding about clinical trials, and at UNC she is leading project PURPLE (Programs to Address Unmet Needs and Promote Representation of All Participants in Lupus Clinical Trials Using Mobile Technology for Engagement). She is actively involved in the education of medical students, residents, subspecialty fellows, and patients.

Lawrence G. Smith, M.D., MACP, is Northwell Health's physician-in-chief. As physician-in-chief, he is Northwell Health's senior physician on all clinical issues. He previously served as Northwell's chief medical officer. Dr. Smith is also the founding dean of the Donald and Barbara Zucker School of Medicine, which received full accreditation by the Liaison Committee on Medical Education and whose first class graduated in May 2015. Dr. Smith joined Northwell in May 2005 as the chief academic officer and the senior vice president of academic affairs. In this capacity, Dr. Smith strengthened Northwell's graduate medical education programs and expanded its medical school affiliations, significantly enhancing Northwell's ability to recruit medical students and residents. In addition, Dr. Smith was responsible for overseeing Northwell's medical student education programs and academic faculty appointments. He was also accountable for establishing close relationships with doctors and hospitals throughout Northwell, which enhanced its partnerships with staff and community-based physicians and improved physician recruitment efforts.

Before joining Northwell, Dr. Smith was at the Icahn School of Medicine at Mount Sinai in Manhattan, where he served as the dean (beginning in 2002) and the chair of medical education, the founder and the director of the school's Institute for Medical Education, a professor of medicine, and an attending physician. He joined the faculty of the Mount Sinai School of Medicine in 1994 as the vice chair of the Department of Medicine and residency program director. Prior to his career at Mount Sinai, Dr. Smith practiced general medicine at Stony Brook University Hospital, where he became a full-time faculty member, the director of education, and the program director of the hospital's residency program in internal medicine. He began his career practicing general internal medicine in Huntington, New York. Dr. Smith has held senior leadership positions in national societies for medical education and residency training, has authored numerous peer-reviewed publications in the area of medical education, and has received many awards and honors from national and international organizations. He is a member-at-large of the National Board of Medical Examiners and is a member of the Board of Visitors of Fordham College. Also, he is a former regent of the American College of Physicians and a former member of the board of directors of the American Board of Internal Medicine. In April 2011, Dr. Smith was elected to Mastership of the American College of Physicians.

Dr. Smith is the first recipient of the Lawrence Scherr, M.D., Professorship of Medicine at the Zucker School of Medicine. He was honored with the 2008 Dema C. Daly Founders Award by the Association of Program Directors of Internal Medicine, of which he is a former president. In addition, he was awarded the Solomon A. Berson Alumni Achievement Award in Health Science by the New York University School of Medicine. Dr. Smith earned a B.S. in physics from Fordham University and an M.D. from the New York University School of Medicine. His residency in internal medicine at Strong Memorial Hospital was followed by military service as a captain in the Army Medical Corps at Fitzsimmons Army Medical Center in Denver.

Patty Spears is a 19-year breast cancer survivor and cancer research advocate. Ms. Spears has extensive clinical trial advocacy experience, having served as an advocate on the Translational Breast Cancer Research Consortium and on the National Cancer Insitute Breast Cancer Steering Committee. She is also an associate group chair for advocacy of the Alliance for Clinical Trials in Oncology (a National Clinical Trial Network group) and the chair of the Alliance Patient Advocate Committee. She is a Komen Scholar, serves as the co-chair on the Komen Advocates in Science Steering Committee, and is a U.S. Food and Drug Administration patient representative. She leads the University of North Carolina (UNC) Lineberger Patient Research Advocacy Group and the UNC Breast Specialized Program of Research Excellence Advocates. At UNC, she focuses on communicating science and clinical research to the public and facilitating the engagement of patients with basic and clinical researchers. She also has an interest in patient-reported outcome measurements in drug development. Ms. Spears is currently working as a scientific research manager and a patient advocate at the UNC Lineberger Comprehensive Cancer Center.

Jovonni R. Spinner, M.P.H., CHES, is a public health strategist and thought leader with a deep passion for improving health equity across the lifespan through research, communication, multisector partnerships, and leadership coaching. She is known as a public health programming guru who uses her skills to direct projects from concept to fully operational through program design, implementation, monitoring, and evaluation, and by breaking down silos across sectors.

At the U.S. Food and Drug Administration (FDA), she is the lead for the outreach and communications team in the Office of Minority Health, where she oversees the strategic direction of the team, advises senior officials on minority health, and leads the Diversity in Clinical Trials Initiative. Prior to joining FDA, she managed national initiatives, including the Community Health Worker Health Disparities Initiative at the National Heart, Lung, and Blood Institute at the National Institutes of Health, which aims to reduce cardiovascular and asthma health disparities through community education and training. She also provided health policy guidance to leaders on vaccine supply and finance policy issues at the U.S. Department of Health and Human Services' National Vaccine Program Office, and served as the director of Virginia's Vaccines for Children Program, ensuring that the state's Medicaid, uninsured, and underinsured populations were vaccinated.

Ms. Spinner serves on nonprofit boards at the American Public University System and the Society for Public Health Education, and writes women's health articles for *Health in Her Hue*. Ms. Spinner received her B.S. in biology from Virginia Commonwealth University, her M.P.H. from the Rollins School of Public Health at Emory University, and is pursuing her Dr.P.H. from Morgan State University.

Alicia Staley is the senior director for patient engagement for mHealth at Medidata. She has more than 20 years of experience in software design and information systems management and works to infuse the patient perspective throughout the product development life cycle and to help engage patients in novel ways.

Ms. Staley is also a three-time cancer survivor, first diagnosed with Hodgkin's disease as a sophomore during college. Over the past 10 years, she has applied her engineering background to improve the patient experience for those dealing with cancer. With an extensive network of patient advocates and nonprofit organizations, she collaborates with a wide range of stakeholders to improve processes and policies that affect patient care and clinical trials. She has co-led several research studies on how patients both share information in online forums and seek out clinical trial opportunities.

An early adopter of social media, she co-founded #BCSM (the Breast Cancer Social Media community), which attracts more than 250 global participants each week to its scheduled online discussions. This foundational online social media support channel is recognized as the gold standard for disease-specific social media networks.

Prior to joining Medidata, Ms. Staley worked at Cure Forward and Science 37, leading their patient recruitment and engagement initiatives to help advance clinical research. As a champion of patient advocacy and engagement, she understands the critical issues facing patients looking to engage in clinical research. With a keen focus on improving access to clinical trials, Ms. Staley is passionate about making a difference for all patients searching for information about clinical trials.

Christopher R. Trudeau, J.D., has a dual appointment at both the University of Arkansas for Medical Sciences (UAMS) and the Bowen School of Law at the University of Arkansas at Little Rock. In his role at Bowen, Professor Trudeau teaches Research, Writing, and Analysis I and II. He has extensive experience teaching legal writing, having taught legal writing to more than 1,500 students during his 13-year tenure at the Western Michigan University–Thomas M. Cooley Law School. While there, Professor Trudeau taught every legal writing course the school offers, and he has become an international leader in plain-language legal writing and drafting. In 2012, Professor Trudeau published the first U.S. study to measure the public's preferences for legal communication, and he has recently received a grant from the Legal Writing Institute, the Association of Legal Writing Directors, and Lexis/Nexis to conduct a similar international study. As an associate professor at the UAMS Center for Health Literacy, he conducts empirical research on clear health communication, drafts health care documents, and teaches health law and communication courses to medical students and students in other health professions. Professor Trudeau is a leading expert on health literacy, informed consent, and risk communication. He often speaks on how to communicate legal and health information in ways that both engage patients and better protect health care organizations. Professor Trudeau frequently speaks on these topics, most recently at the Centers for Disease Control and Prevention, the U.S. Food and Drug Administration, and the National Academies of Sciences, Engineering, and Medicine.

Consuelo H. Wilkins, M.D., MSCI, is the recently appointed vice president for health equity at the Vanderbilt University Medical Center and is the associate dean for health equity at the Vanderbilt University School of Medicine. Dr. Wilkins is a clinical investigator and an engagement researcher who is an associate director of the Vanderbilt Institute for Clinical and Translational Science, where she oversees programs in community engagement and team science. Dr. Wilkins is a principal investigator of the Vanderbilt-Miami-Meharry Center of Excellence in Precision Medicine and Population Health, which focuses on decreasing disparities among African Americans and Latinos using precision medicine, and at the Vanderbilt Recruitment Innovation Center, a national center dedicated to enhancing recruitment and retention in clinical trials. She is widely recognized for her innovative work on developing and testing methods and tools to engage patients and communities in research. She serves as the director of the Engagement Core of the All of Us Research Program, a national precision-medicine project that will enroll 1 million or more participants. In the interim, Dr. Wilkins also continues to serve as the executive director of the Meharry–Vanderbilt Alliance. She holds faculty appointments as an associate professor of medicine at both the Vanderbilt University Medical Center and Meharry Medical College. Prior to her current roles, Dr. Wilkins was an associate professor in the Department of Medicine, Division of Geriatrics, with secondary appointments in psychiatry and surgery (Public Health Sciences) at the Washington University School of Medicine in St. Louis. She served as the founding director of the Center for Community Health and Partnerships in the Institute for Public Health, the co-director of the Center for Community Engaged Research in the Clinical Translational Science Awards, and the co-founder of Our Community, Our Health, a collaborative program with St. Louis University, to disseminate culturally relevant health information and facilitate community–academic partnerships to address health disparities.

Rebecca J. Williams, Pharm.D., M.P.H., is the acting director at Clinical Trials.gov at the National Center for Biotechnology Information, National Library of Medicine, National Institutes of Health in Bethesda, Maryland. She moved into this role after serving as the assistant director of ClinicalTrials.gov for more than a decade. She is responsible for technical, scientific, policy, regulatory, and outreach activities related to the operation of ClinicalTrials.gov, an international registry-and-results database of clinical research. Her research interests relate to improving the quality of reporting for clinical research. Her prior experience includes serving as a regulatory affairs consultant and a reviewer and in supervisory roles at the U.S. Food and Drug Administration in the area of prescription drug advertising and promotion. She received her Pharm.D. from the University of Wisconsin–Madison and her M.P.H. from the Bloomberg School of Public Health at Johns Hopkins University.